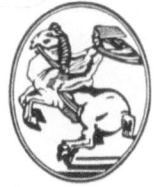

VIROLOGY
MONOGRAPHS

DIE VIRUSFORSCHUNG
IN EINZELDARSTELLUNGEN

CONTINUATION OF / FORTFÜHRUNG VON
HANDBOOK OF VIRUS RESEARCH
HANDBUCH DER VIRUSFORSCHUNG
FOUNDED BY / BEGRÜNDET VON
R. DOERR

EDITED BY / HERAUSGEGEBEN VON

S. GARD · C. HALLAUER

16

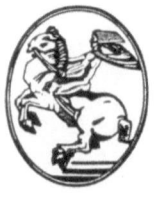

SPRINGER-VERLAG
WIEN NEW YORK

DENGUE VIRUSES

BY

R. W. SCHLESINGER

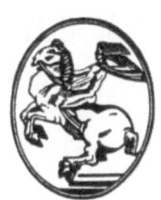

SPRINGER-VERLAG

WIEN NEW YORK

Softcover reprint of the hardcover 1st edition 1977

Library of Congress Cataloging in Publication Data. Schlesinger, Robert Walter, 1913—. Dengue viruses.
(Virology monographs; 16.) Bibliography: p. 1. Dengue viruses. I. Title. II. Series. QR360. V52. no. 16
[QR398]. 576'.64'08s [616.01'94]. 77–24108

ISBN-13: 978-3-7091-8468-4   e-ISBN-13: 978-3-7091-8466-0
DOI:10.1007/978-3-7091-8466-0

Dengue Viruses

By

R. Walter Schlesinger

Department of Microbiology, College of Medicine and Dentistry of New Jersey,
Rutgers Medical School,
Piscataway, New Jersey

With the collaboration of **S. Hotta**

Department of Microbiology, Kobe University, School of Medicine,
Kobe, Japan

With 34 Figures

Preface

This monograph is dedicated to the memory of ROBERT DOERR (1871—1951), the founder of the Handbuch der Virusforschung which was the predecessor of this series of Virology Monographs. In 1939, he also founded the Archiv für die gesamte Virusforschung, the first journal devoted to virology. His comprehensive vision, expressed in these publications, marked him as a father of modern virology as a distinct science. The tradition established by him was ably continued by his long-time collaborator and editorial successor, CURT HALLAUER, with whom I share the privilege of having been introduced to viruses by DOERR.

More specifically, the subject of this monograph was one of personal interest to DOERR. His studies of sandfly (pappataci) fever stand as a classical demonstration of the role of arthropods in the transmission of human virus diseases[1,2] and led him to write an authoritative review of that disease and of dengue[3].

During the second World War, Japanese and American investigators independently succeeded in propagating dengue virus in mice and in developing attenuated strains suitable for experimental vaccination of human subjects. Professor S. HOTTA, now at Kobe University, was a member of the Japanese team. He and his associates have continued to make valuable contributions to dengue research. I worked with the group led by Dr. ALBERT B. SABIN in the United States. When I was asked by Professor HALLAUER to write this monograph, I invited Professor HOTTA to be a coauthor. In 1968, he supplied valuable references and summaries, many pertaining to work published in Japan to which I did not have access. Unfortunately, various distractions forced me to postpone my own writing, and the

---

[1] DOERR, R., FRANZ, K., TAUSSIG, S.: Das Pappatacifieber. Leipzig-Wien: Deuticke 1909.

[2] DOERR, R., RUSS, V. K.: Weitere Untersuchungen über das Pappatacifieber. Arch. für Schiffs- und Tropen-Hygiene **13**, 693—706 (1909).

[3] DOERR, R.: Pappatacifieber und Dengue, in: Handbuch der pathogenen Mikroorganismen (KOLLE, WASSERMANN, eds.), pp. 500—546. Jena: Fischer 1930.

1

rapid flow of new knowledge made sustained long-distance coauthorship virtually impossible. The resulting delays compelled Professor HOTTA to meet deadlines in the publication of his book "Dengue and Related Hemorrhagic Diseases" (St.Louis: W. H. Green, Inc. 1969). In order to avoid duplication. the emphasis of this monograph had to be re-oriented. Professor HOTTA graciously agreed to change coauthorship to an acknowledgment of our early collaboration in portions of the text. The greater part represents my reflections and interpretations for which Professor HOTTA should not be held responsible. I am grateful for his contributions and understanding.

Most of the text was written and re-written during brief periods of undisturbed quiet at the Rockefeller Foundation's Study and Conference Center, Bellagio, Italy (October 1972), and at the Library of the Marine Biological Laboratory, Woods Hole, Massachusetts.

Piscataway, N.J., March 1977 R. WALTER SCHLESINGER

Table of Contents

I. Introduction

Dengue fever is a mosquito-transmitted disease of man which has afflicted untold millions of people over the past two centuries. It is caused by viruses classified as a subgroup of the group B togaviruses. Along with other members of that group as well as group A, the dengue viruses have been investigated intensively during recent years. Certain unique aspects of their structure, composition, antigenicity, replication, and antigenic relationships have established the togavirus family as quite distinct from other families of enveloped RNA viruses (see recent review of PFEFFERKORN and SHAPIRO, 1974). The basic studies leading to this conclusion have coincided with epidemiological field investigations which have resulted in a continuing increase in the number of viruses now designated as group A or B togaviruses. This, in turn, has led to a growing appreciation of their immense importance as actual or potential pathogens of man and beast.

All group A togaviruses (or alphaviruses) are antigenically and structurally related to each other, yet each one has its own antigenic and biological specificity. The same is true for group B togaviruses (or flaviviruses). Most viruses now unequivocally classified as togaviruses (cf. HORZINEK, 1973 a, b) are also arthropod-borne (arbo)viruses, *i.e.*, they are transmitted to vertebrate hosts by arthropod vectors in which they multiply and establish life-long infection (cf. BERGE, 1975). What is the evolutionary significance of this infection cycle? What are the selective pressures that such a complex, apparently mandatory, alternation between invertebrate and vertebrate hosts imposes on viruses? What are the consequences of these pressures in terms of antigenic and pathogenic variation? These are among the questions for which carefully designed laboratory models may ultimately provide some answers.

In addition to the dengue viruses, group B contains some 50 other viruses. Although logic might suggest that a monograph ought to cover all of them rather than just the dengue subgroup, we know very little about many members of the group. A few—notably Japanese, Murray Valley, and St. Louis encephalitis (JE, MVE, SLE), Kunjin, certain tick-borne encephalitis (TBE) viruses—have been analyzed to about the same extent as dengue viruses. By and large, the information obtained is remarkably similar for all of them. Comparative data will be included in this monograph whenever they supplement in essential detail our knowledge about dengue viruses.

Why then have the dengue viruses been selected as the subject for this monograph? One reason is purely historical. Dengue fever was the second specifically *human* disease (after yellow fever) whose etiology was critically identified as a "filtrable virus" (ASHBURN and CRAIG, 1907). Immense efforts were made subsequently to learn more about the disease and its epidemiology and to make the virus amenable to laboratory investigation. This work was summarized in the classical monographs by SILER *et al.* (1926) and SIMMONS *et al.* (1931). In the decade immediately preceding World War II, however, the importance of dengue was eclipsed by that of its close relative, yellow fever, and by the success in development of an effective YF vaccine (see STRODE, 1951). The Pacific phase of World War II brought dengue fever to renewed prominence, and that era signified a beginning of the detailed knowledge about dengue viruses and the diseases they cause that we have now acquired. Therefore this seems to be a good time to amplify earlier résumés of the work accomplished in the 1940's and 1950's (SABIN, 1952a, d; HOTTA, 1965, 1969).

Like yellow fever, dengue has a relatively simple transmission cycle which involves only certain species of mosquitoes and man (and occasionally monkeys). In this respect these two viruses differ from most other serious pathogens in the group, notably the encephalitis viruses, which have a far more complex transmission cycle and for which man is a relatively minor, accidental, or dead-end link. Moreover, while these latter viruses do infect man in nature, the vast majority of human infections remain subclinical.

In contrast, a first infection with one of the dengue viruses almost invariably leads to some kind of illness. Man, being the single major natural host, is bound to reflect in his response to infection any variable property of the viruses that may affect their pathogenicity. The fact that exposure to one virus of the dengue subgroup may profoundly modify the immunopathological response to subsequent infection with another one has, in recent years, forced us dramatically to change our earlier view of dengue fever as a benign disease. The more alarming aspect of dengue viruses has emerged by virtue of their documented association with "new" and often fatal illnesses, *i.e.*, hemorrhagic fever and the dengue shock syndrome (HAMMON, 1969; HAMMON *et al.*, 1957, 1958, 1960a, b; cf. HALSTEAD, 1965, 1966). Current hypotheses explain the pathogenesis of these syndromes by taking into account known or surmised aspects of the structural and antigenic nature of the viruses, the mode of their replication and release from infected cells, and the host's immune response.

A major difficulty in summarizing information about on "old" virus disease lies in the fact that many classical studies have been rendered obsolete or questionable by more recent findings. The monumental review of dengue by SILER, HALL, and HITCHENS (1926) contains nearly 600 literature references, many of them of fascinating historical interest. It would go beyond the scope of this monograph to sort out those which seem relevant in light of current ideas.

More recent epidemiological data on dengue are represented in a vast literature reporting the results of mass surveys of human and animal populations or of potential arthropod vectors for serological or virological evidence of infection with many different kinds of arboviruses (cf. THEILER and DOWNS, 1973). The main contribution of this approach is the elucidation of the overall prevalence of arboviruses and, specifically, of ecological factors which may be responsible for the emergence of a seemingly endless variety of species among these agents. Its value has been underlined by the recent recognition that a great majority of arboviruses not previously accommodated in the togavirus groups can in fact be fitted into a third large family, the bunyaviruses (MURPHY et al., 1973; PORTERFIELD et al., 1974; BERGE, 1975). Thus, it seems that the biological feature of arthropod-vertebrate-arthropod- ... transmission cycles is frequently associated with viruses belonging to two major structural families, the toga- and bunyaviruses.

Table 1. *Selected fever epidemics by year,*

Present-day chikungunya (? original dengue)
(Fever, joint pain, rash, residual arthralgias)

Year	Location	Designation
1779	Batavia	Knuckle fever
1779	Cairo	Knee trouble
1823	Zanzibar	Dinga, dyenga
1824—25	Calcutta; Madras; Gujarat	Scarletina rheumatica
1827 –28	West Indies, New Orleans; Charleston, S.C.	Dandy fever, eruptive articular fever, exanthesis arthrosia, dengue
1870	Zanzibar	Dinga, dyenga, dengue
1871—72	Calcutta; Madras	Dengue
1901– 02	Hong Kong; Burma; Madras	Dengue
1923	Calcutta	Dengue
1952	Tanganyika	Chikungunya (prototype virus isolated)
1964	Vellore, India	Chinkungunya (virus isolated)

From CAREY (1971). With permission of the author and the Journal of the History of Medicine.

This circumstance alone carries fascinating implications regarding possible parallels in their evolutionary history (cf. SCHLESINGER, 1971). Within the broad spectrum of the 200-odd viruses so far assigned to these families, the dengue virus subgroup presents unique features.

In this monograph we shall concentrate on knowledge about dengue viruses gained since the second World War, when they first became amenable to intensive study in the laboratory.

II. Definitions and Nomenclature

Dengue is the accepted name of an acute infectious disease of man characterized by fever, aches and pains in various parts of the body which may range from mild to excruciatingly severe, generalized rash, lymphadenopathy and leukopenia. Its effects may be debilitating to the point of prostration, but uncomplicated classical

location, symptomatology, and designation

	Present-day dengue (? original breakbone) (Diphasic fever, body and muscle pain, rash, post-illness asthenia)	
Year	Location	Designation
1780	Philadelphia	Breakbone fever
1826—27	Charleston, S.C.; Savannah, Ga.	Breakbone fever
1850	Charleston, S.C.	Breakbone fever
1853—54	Calcutta	(loin and limb pain, languor, prostration. Only one case with severe articular pain)
1897	Queensland, Australia	Dengue
1905	Queensland, Australia	Dengue (transmission via *A. aegypti* shown)
1905—07	Calcutta	Seven day fever
1907	Philippines	Dengue (transmitted via filtered plasma)
1907	Brownsville, Tex.	Dengue
1911—12	Calcutta; Poona	Seven-day fever, dengue
1923	Galveston, Tex.	Dengue
1944—45	Hawaii, New Guinea; Calcutta	Dengue (prototype viruses isolated)
1961—63	Vellore, India	Dengue (viruses isolated)

(primary) dengue is rarely, if ever, fatal. It is caused by at least four antigenically distinct viruses constituting the dengue subgroup of group B togaviruses (see Section IV on Classification). By definition, they are transmitted to man by mosquitoes of the genus *Aedes* (Stegomyia). It follows that the occurrence of the disease (and the viruses) is restricted to those geographic areas in which suitable vector species are prevalent or in which, once imported, they can maintain themselves.

Virus can be isolated from the peripheral blood of naturally infected patients during the febrile phase of the acute disease (cf. SABIN. 1952a). In the past, it had to be identified by its ability to produce typical dengue in human subjects inoculated by a variety of routes or bitten by *Aedes* mosquitoes which had engorged on virus-containing source material (SILER *et al.*, 1926). Since the first successful experimental transmissions of dengue viruses to mice (KIMURA and HOTTA, 1944; SABIN and SCHLESINGER, 1945; MEIKLEJOHN *et al.*, 1952a; SCHLESINGER and FRANKEL, 1952a), this method and the use of various *in vitro* cell cultures, in combination with serological and physical-chemical criteria, have been applied to their primary isolation and identification (see subsequent sections).

The origin of the name dengue has been puzzling. According to HALSTEAD (1971), the word may have its roots in the Swahili term "ki-denga Pepo" or "a disease characterized by the sudden cramp-like seizure caused by an evil spirit", which was applied to an outbreak in Zanzibar in 1870. "The term 'denga' or 'dyenga' was used to designate the disease on the East Coast of Africa in 1823 and at least until 1870. Early authors have assumed that 'dengue' spread with the slave trade from East Africa to the Caribbean. where in 1827—28 an extensive outbreak occurred in the West Indies . . . It was here that the word dengue was first used", perhaps as a Spanish adaptation of the imported word. Although it now appears that the illness to which African natives referred as "denga" etc. may actually have been *chikungunya* (CAREY, 1971; HALSTEAD, 1971a; see next Section), it is now of course possible to distinguish these two diseases by virological and serological means. As might be expected for a disease as painful, wide-spread, and old as dengue, many exotic and picturesque synonyms have been in circulation at various times and places (fully discussed by SILER *et al.*, 1926, and by CAREY. 1971, see Table 1). The colloquial "breakbone fever" is a very apt and descriptive term.

III. History

The early history of "dengue", going back to epidemics in Java and in Egypt in 1779, was admirably reviewed by SILER *et al.* (1926). These authors quoted extensively from old documents to support their hypothesis that dengue had occurred in the Western hemisphere as early as the mid-17th century and had its origin in "tropical America" (l. c., p. 21). On the other hand, MATTINGLY (1960) summarized evidence which led him to believe that it originated in Southeast Asia.

A recent scholarly treatise by CAREY (1971) analyzed critically the historical accounts of "dengue" outbreaks during the 18th and 19th century. CAREY furnished persuasive arguments in favor of the belief that the earliest recorded epidemics outside the Western hemisphere (including those in Java, Egypt and India) were probably due to chikungunya virus (a group A togavirus) rather than dengue viruses. Table 1, taken from CAREY's paper, summarizes the key differences in clinical characteristics and assigns various epidemics to one or the other of the two agents.

We owe to BENJAMIN RUSH the first accurate clinical description of true dengue fever as it occurred during the Philadelphia epidemic of 1780 (quoted in SILER *et al.*, 1926, and CAREY, 1971). It fits, in many details, the features of the disease seen in well-documented contemporary outbreaks (see Section X).

During the 19th and 20th centuries, extensive outbreaks were reported from tropical and subtropical areas on all continents and from many subcontinents and islands in the South Pacific and in the Caribbean. This extensive geographic spread has continued to the present day. For example, during this century major epidemics were recorded in the Southern United States (1920, 1922), Australia (1925—26, 1942, 1954—55), South Africa (1926—27), Greece (1927—28), Japan (1942—45), and the Caribbean (1963—69). The occurrence of dengue in the Caribbean during the past decade is illustrated in Figs. 1—4. Its relationship to the prevalence of *Aedes aegypti* is clearly shown in Fig. 4.

Each of these epidemics affected thousands or millions of people, with disease rates in some areas attaining 80% of the population (*e.g.*, COPANARIS, 1928, who reported that 80—90% of the populace of Athens and Piraeus contracted dengue during the Greek epidemic). Such massive outbreaks, even those occurring at a time when methods for virus isolation or serological diagnosis were not available, have aided greatly in the delineation of clinical and epidemiological features of the disease. This was particularly true for the outbreaks in South Africa, the United States, Greece and Japan because these areas have experienced no major subsequent occurrence. As a result, it has been possible, through retrospective serological surveys, to support the view that these epidemics were indeed caused by dengue viruses (KOKERNOT *et al.*, 1956; SIGEL and BEASLEY, 1959; HAMMON *et al.*, 1966; EHRENKRANZ *et al.*, 1971; THEILER *et al.*, 1960; PAVLATOS and SMITH, 1964; HOTTA, 1968; HOTTA *et al.*, 1968). As discussed in detail by WISSEMAN and SWEET (1961) and WISSEMAN (1961), this type of circumstantial confirmation is extremely important in view of the fact that the dengue syndrome is mimicked by a variety of other agents, including several other arthropod-transmitted viruses. Moreover, not all epidemics of verified dengue display the disease in its full-blown incapacitating form; occasionally relatively mild, easily confused variations predominate. Mild forms are particularly characteristic in childhood when most people are likely to acquire their first infection in heavily endemic areas (*e.g.*, Southeast Asia) (cf. HALSTEAD *et al.*, 1969b) (see Section X). In "hyperendemic" areas (Haiti and Dominican Republic), clinical illness may be completely absent (VENTURA *et al.*, 1975). Therefore, estimates of the geographic distribution of the disease or its viruses strictly on the basis of clinical evaluation of epidemic or sporadic occurrences of "dengue" or "dengue-like" disease are somewhat precarious. Again, the situation has been clarified to some extent by CAREY (1971). His searching review of the earlier literature leads to the conclusion that the distinction between "dengue" (*i.e.*, chikungunya) and "seven-day fever" or "breakbone fever" (*i.e.*, dengue by current designation) was indeed made by some astute

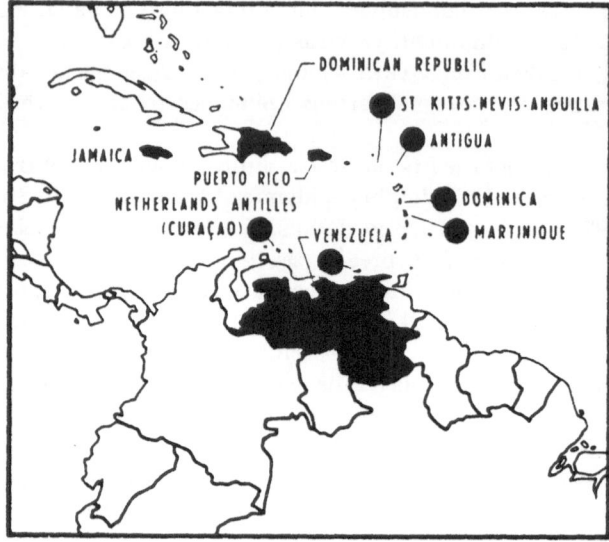

Fig. 1

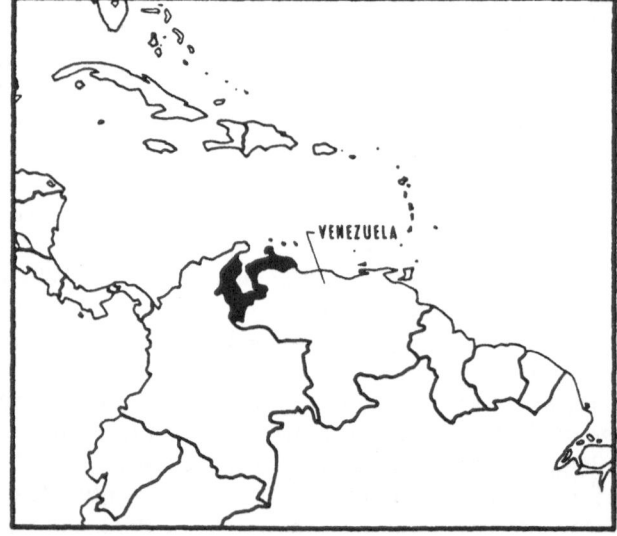

Fig. 2

Fig. 1. Occurrence of dengue in the Caribbean, 1963—1965
Fig. 2. Occurrence of dengue in the Caribbean, 1966—1967
Fig. 3. Occurrence of dengue in the Caribbean, 1968—1969
Fig. 4. Status of the aedes aegypti eradication campaign in the Americas,
December 1969

Figs. 1—4. From "Surveillance of Dengue in the Americas: A Report to the Director",
Pan American Health Organization, Report of the Scientific Advisory Committee on
Dengue, First Meeting 15—16 January 1970
With permission of The Pan American Health Organization

DOMINICAN REPUBLIC
HAITI
ST. KITTS-NEVIS-ANGUILLA
ANTIGUA
MONTSERRAT
DOMINICA
BARBADOS
ST. LUCIA
ST. VINCENT
GRENADA
JAMAICA
PUERTO RICO
VENEZUELA

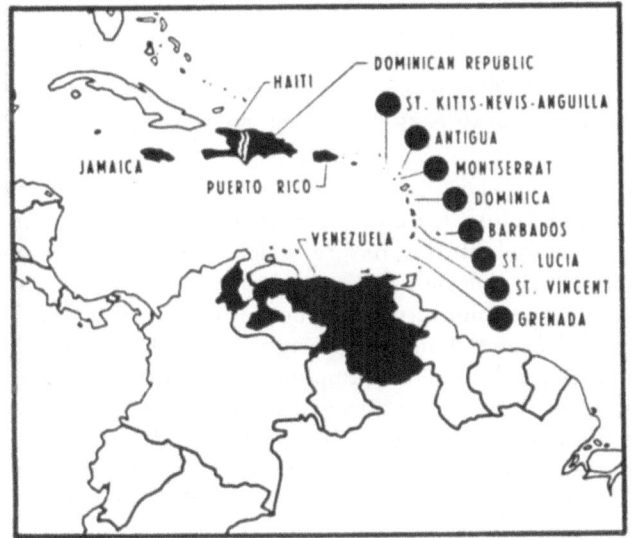

Fig. 3

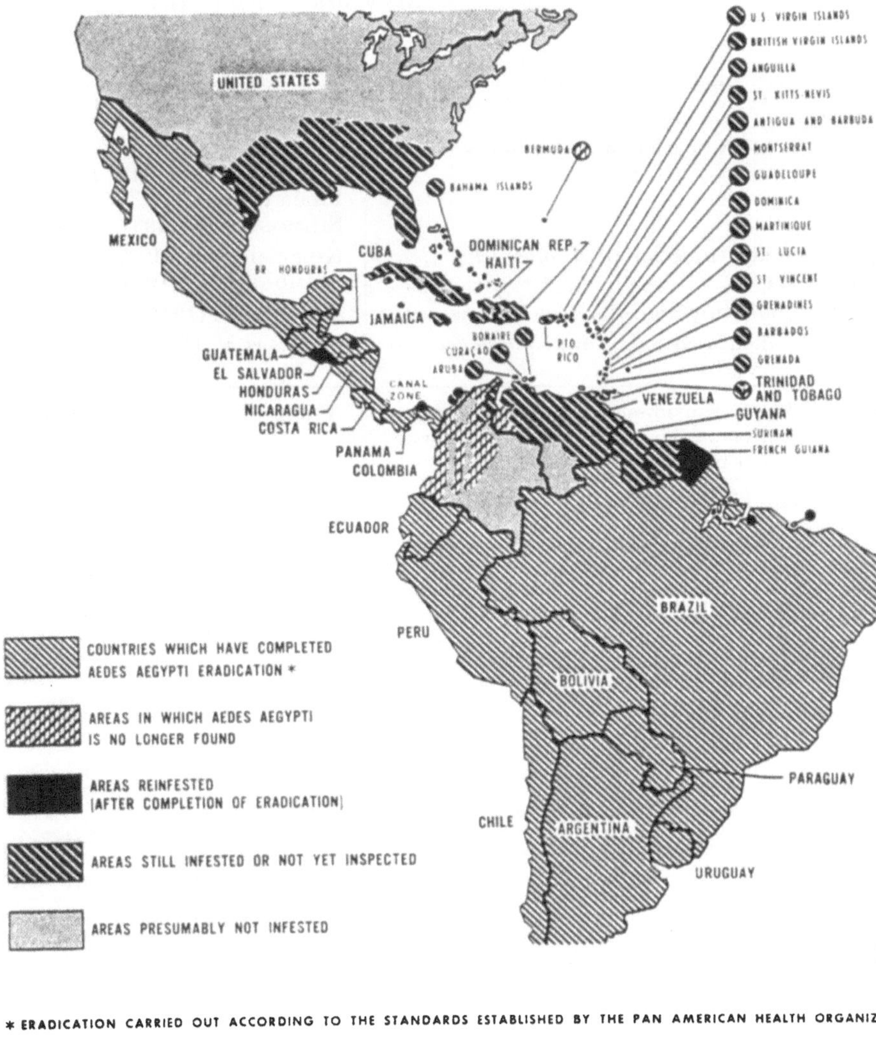
UNITED STATES
BERMUDA
BAHAMA ISLANDS
MEXICO
CUBA
DOMINICAN REP.
HAITI
BR. HONDURAS
JAMAICA
BONAIRE
CURAÇAO
ARUBA
PTO RICO
GUATEMALA
EL SALVADOR
HONDURAS
NICARAGUA
COSTA RICA
CANAL ZONE
PANAMA
COLOMBIA
VENEZUELA
U.S. VIRGIN ISLANDS
BRITISH VIRGIN ISLANDS
ANGUILLA
ST. KITTS-NEVIS
ANTIGUA AND BARBUDA
MONTSERRAT
GUADELOUPE
DOMINICA
MARTINIQUE
ST. LUCIA
ST. VINCENT
GRENADINES
BARBADOS
GRENADA
TRINIDAD AND TOBAGO
GUYANA
SURINAM
FRENCH GUIANA
ECUADOR
BRAZIL
PERU
BOLIVIA
PARAGUAY
CHILE
ARGENTINA
URUGUAY
COUNTRIES WHICH HAVE COMPLETED AEDES AEGYPTI ERADICATION *
AREAS IN WHICH AEDES AEGYPTI IS NO LONGER FOUND
AREAS REINFESTED (AFTER COMPLETION OF ERADICATION)
AREAS STILL INFESTED OR NOT YET INSPECTED
AREAS PRESUMABLY NOT INFESTED

Fig. 4

* ERADICATION CARRIED OUT ACCORDING TO THE STANDARDS ESTABLISHED BY THE PAN AMERICAN HEALTH ORGANIZATION

early clinicians (see Table 1). The differences between the two diseases, as they have been observed in recent outbreaks, have been summarized by DELLER and RUSSELL (1967).

In the evolution of knowledge about dengue and similar illnesses, military exigencies have traditionally provided a major spur. One obvious reason for this interest is, of course, their debilitating nature which can render combat forces ineffective (cf. McCoy, 1964). Another factor is the massive transfer, in war or peace, of previously unexposed military personnel into endemic areas. Thus, an early entry of the United States Army into dengue research was forced by the experience that troops shipped to the Philippine Islands inevitably contracted the disease even though native Scouts, garrisoned alongside, did not. This remarkable contrast led to the first controlled studies on immunity to dengue (SILER et al., 1926; SIMMONS et al., 1931; see also the recent follow-up on their studies by HALSTEAD, 1975). Again, the Pacific phase of World War II confronted both

Table 2. *Summary of "classical" studies of dengue and its viruses*

Subject	References
A. *Transmission by mosquitoes*	GRAHAM (1903)
(a) Specific identification of *A. aegypti* as vector	BANCROFT (1906)
	CLELAND *et al.* (1916, 1919)
	SILER *et al.* (1926)
	SIMMONS *et al.* (1931)
(b) Specific identification of *A. albopictus* as vector	KOIZUMI *et al.* (1916)
	SIMMONS *et al.* (1931)
(c) Specific identification of *A. scutellaris* as vector	MACKERRAS (1946)
(d) Specific identification of *A. polynesiensis* Marks as vector	ROSEN *et al.* (1954)
B. *Viral etiology* (transmission by inoculation of human volunteers with infectious human plasma passed through bacteria-retaining filters)	ASHBURN and CRAIG (1907)
C. *Experimental demonstration of immunity to reinfection*	SILER *et al.* (1926)
	SIMMONS *et al.* (1931)
D. *Experimental infection of monkeys*	BLANC *et al.* (1929)
E. *Propagation in mice and attenuation of human pathogenicity*	KIMURA and HOTTA (1944)
	SABIN and SCHLESINGER (1945)
F. *Multiple immunologic types*	
(a) Types 1 and 2	SABIN and SCHLESINGER (1945)
	SABIN (1950)
(b) Types 3 and 4	HAMMON *et al.* (1960a, b)
G. *Immunologic relationship to other group B arboviruses*	SABIN (1950)
	CASALS and BROWN (1954)
H. *Propagation in tissue culture*	HOTTA and EVANS (1956a, b)
I. *Role of dengue viruses in Southeast Asian hemorrhagic fevers*	HAMMON *et al.* (1960a, b)

Japan and the United States with the potential hazards of combat in dengue endemic areas and stimulated renewed efforts in both countries to investigate the disease and its causative agent (cf. SABIN, 1952a; HOTTA, 1965, 1969).

The success of these studies was directly responsible for the specific identification of epidemic and endemic dengue in various parts of the world and for the unequivocal demonstration that dengue viruses are causally related to hemorrhagic fevers and the shock syndrome in South and Southeast Asia (HAMMON *et al.*, 1960a, b). The latter alarming development has provided renewed stimulus to dissect the virion physically and biochemically, to study its antigenic components, and to understand the pathogenesis of primary and secondary disease in terms of current pathophysiological and immunological concepts.

Some initial contributions to major phases of dengue virus research are summarized in Table 2. From the point of view of facilitating accumulation of knowledge about the basic properties of dengue viruses, their "adaptation" to the laboratory mouse was the crucial step. It permitted, for the first time, the circumvention of man as the only available experimental host, facilitated the eventual propagation and quantitation of the viruses in *in vitro* cell cultures, and led to advances in their physical, antigenic, and biochemical characterization.

IV. Classification

Remarkable passages from a paper by OSGOOD (1828), commenting on an outbreak of "dengue" in Havana, Cuba, are quoted by CAREY (1971): "The people of Havana have named this strange fever 'El Dengue' which word signifies, literally, affectation ... The dengues has, as yet, only prevailed in the places to which the yellow fever has been limited. It has not spread to the interior of Cuba, although, at the end of five months from the time of its rise in Havana, it continues to attack most of the persons who come to the city from the country ... *I have been led to consider the specific cause of the disease of the present time, and that of the yellow fever, to be the same.* The subjects have become altered in their constitutions; but the generating cause both of the new and the old fever remains unchanged." Although CAREY assigns the West Indian outbreak to the chikungunya category (Table 1), this early hint at epidemiological coincidence is no less striking.

Almost one-hundred years later, SILER *et al.* (1926) wrote: "Attention has been repeatedly called to the several striking points of similarity between dengue and yellow fever. Noteworthy among the contributions which have discussed the factors in which the two diseases are practically identical are those of CRAIG (1911, 1920). *This author is of the opinion that the etiologic agent of dengue, when it is found, will prove to belong to the same group as does that of yellow fever.*"

The validity of these empirical prophecies, based on clinical-epidemiological considerations, was verified in 1950, when SABIN reported cross-reactions of human dengue-convalescent sera not only with yellow fever (YF) but also with Japanese B encephalitis (JBE) and West Nile (WN) antigens. Subsequently, it was shown by CASALS and BROWN (1954) that a variety of arthropod-borne viruses could be categorized into two major groups (A and B) on the basis of (a) optimal conditions required for hemagglutination (HA) (see Section V.B.2.), and (b) cross-reactivity in hemagglutination-inhibition (HI) tests (see Section VI, E). According to both criteria, dengue viruses belonged to group B, along with JE. Ilheus, Ntaya, Russian spring-summer encephalitis (RSSE), St. Louis encephalitis (SLE), WN, and YF viruses. Later studies by CASALS and coworkers led to the establishment of several other groups of arthropod-borne viruses on the basis of major or minor serological cross-reactions. The list of those assigned to group B has grown to 57 (BERGE, 1975), making it the second largest of the arbovirus groups [the largest being the Bunyavirus family (BERGE, 1975)] and the one containing the largest number (29) of proved human pathogens.

According to the recommendations of a WHO Study Group (WHO, 1967), the criteria for acceptance of an arthropod-borne virus should be as follows: "Arbo-viruses are viruses which are maintained in nature principally, or to an important extent, through biological transmission between susceptible vertebrate hosts by haematophagous arthropods; they multiply and produce viraemia in the vertebrates, multiply in the tissues of arthropods, and are passed on to new vertebrates by the bites of arthropods after a period of extrinsic incubation."

In recent years, the group designations (A, B, C, etc.) were amplified by generic names, e.g., "alphavirus" for group A, "flavivirus" (*flavus* for yellow fever) for group B (cf. WILDY, 1971). Various other amplifying suggestions for the refinement of a classification of arboviruses on purely biological grounds have been debated (SCHERER, 1968; CASALS, 1968a; JOHNSON, 1968; TAURASO and SHELOKOV, 1967). We shall follow SCHERER's suggestion (1968) to regard the four generally accepted, serologically distinct, dengue viruses as types 1, 2, 3, and 4 (hereafter referred to as dengue-1, -2, -3, -4) of the dengue subgroup of group B arboviruses (flaviviruses). This designation takes account of the fact that these 4 types (a) share the biological characteristics generally associated with dengue viruses (clinical features, epi-demiology, natural and experimental host range, vector specificity), (b) possess type-specific antigens, (c) carry, in addition, some as yet unexplained subgroup-specific antigenic relationships, but (d) share antigenic determinant(s) with all group B arboviruses.

The term "arbovirus", by etymological derivation as well as by definition, implies nothing more than a convenient collection bag for viruses meeting the biological criteria cited above. The need for a more discriminating assignment of the different groups and members to a rational system of viruses based on physical-chemical properties (LWOFF and TOURNIER, 1966; GIBBS and HARRISON, 1968; WILDY, 1971) has been stressed by JOHNSON (1968). It is underlined by the confusing (but understandable) proposal to classify rubella virus as an arbovirus (HOLMES and WARBURTON, 1967; HOLMES et al., 1969) on the grounds that it resembles certain group A arboviruses in physical-chemical characteristics and in features of its mode of replication and release. While the absence of serological cross reactions between rubella or other structurally similar viruses (cf. HORZINEK, 1973a, b) and a large number of arboviruses (METTLER et al., 1968) does not seem an adequate basis for rejecting a systematic relationship (after all, arthropod trans-mission *could* be an ecologic accident and lack of it *could* be an evolutionary adaptation; moreover, different *groups* of arboviruses also are completely unrelated serologically), the known biological features of rubella, LDH virus and others do rule out their designation as arthropod-borne, *i.e.*, arboviruses.

It was initially proposed by LWOFF and TOURNIER (1966) that the dilemma of the proper classification of arboviruses be resolved by coining the family name *Togaviridae* for those viruses sufficiently characterized in terms of physical-chemical characteristics and patterns of replication to fit them into the LWOFF-TOURNIER system as a homogeneous order. This proposal has now been sanctioned by the International Committee on Nomenclature of Viruses (WILDY, 1971; MELNICK, 1973; FENNER, 1976), and, accordingly, the term group B togavirus will be used here to describe the genus to which the dengue viruses belong. Table 3 summarizes the properties which dengue viruses share with other well-studied members of the genus and which will be documented in detail in the appropriate sections below. Thus, in terms of the cryptograms proposed by GIBBS *et al.* (1966, 1968), the properties of the dengue viruses are R/1:4.2/7:S/*:V, I/Di.

Table 3. *Properties of dengue viruses*

1. *Physical-chemical*	
a. Virion structure	Spherical, enveloped, ~500 Å diameter; envelope carries knob-like projections; central "core" ~250 Å diameter, roughly hexagonal in cross-section; nucleocapsid of uncertain symmetry.
b. Genome	Linear ss-RNA; 45 S; MW ~4.2×10^6 daltons; U = 22, G = 26, C = 21, A = 31.
c. Structural proteins	At least 3 polypeptides: VP 1, MW ~8,000, assoc. with envelope; VP 2, MW ~13,000, assoc. with RNA (nucleocapsid protein); VP 3, MW ~59,000, glycoprotein assoc. with envelope.
d. Lipids	Present in envelope.
2. *Replication*	In cytoplasm; only traces of "replicative intermediate" RNase-sensitive, ~26 S RNA; RNase-resistant ~20 S dsRF-RNA; only prelim. data on RNA polymerase which is said to produce 20—26 S heterodisperse ss-RNA; 140 S RNP "cores" in cytoplasm; assembly and release of virions prob. associated with cytoplasmic membranes.
3. *Metabolic inhibitors*	Not inhibited by actinomycin D, guanidine-HCl; inhibited by 5-fluorouridine, 6-azauridine, puromycin.
4. *Biological properties*	
a. Host range	Natural: Man, monkeys, *Aedes* mosquitoes.
	Experimental: Man, monkeys, mice, chick embryos; various primary or established cell cultures of human, simian, porcine, rodent, avian, mosquito origins.
b. Hemagglutination	Certain avian erythrocytes; pH-dependent
5. *Antigens*	*Group*-specific (*i.e.*, shared by all group B togaviruses) assoc. with nucleocapsid.
	Subgroup- (*i.e.*, dengue) and *type*- (*i.e.*, dengue-1, -2, -3, -4) specific assoc. with envelope, probably VP 3 glycoprotein. In addition, infected cells produce a non-structural protein, MW ~39,000, which carries subgroup- and type-specific Ag determinants.

V. Biological Systems Used to Study Basic Viral Properties

Before proceeding to a review of physical and chemical studies on dengue viruses, it may be helpful to describe briefly the host systems used to obtain virus for experimental work and assay procedures for monitoring virus-specific biological activities.

A. Host Systems Serving as Sources of Virus

1. Man

The dependence of early dengue research on the availability of human subjects has already been mentioned. Until 1944, human serum, obtained during the acute phase of infection, was the only reliable source of virus for experimental work. It was used to demonstrate the following: (1) presence of filtrable virus in blood (ASHBURN and CRAIG, 1907; CLELAND et al., 1919; SABIN, 1952a), (2) concentration of virus in acute phase blood equivalent of at least 2×10^6 (KOIZUMI et al., 1916) or 1×10^6 (SABIN, 1952a) (see also ROSEN and GUBLER, 1974) human infectious doses per milliliter; (3) existence of multiple antigenic types (SABIN and SCHLESIN-GER, 1945; SABIN, 1950; HAMMON et al., 1960a, b); (4) infectivity for monkeys (BLANC et al., 1929; BLANC and CAMINOPETROS, 1930; SIMMONS et al., 1931; FINDLAY, 1932; also later studies discussed in sections on Experimental Infection and Immunization), mice (KIMURA and HOTTA, 1944a; SABIN and SCHLESINGER, 1945; MEIKLEJOHN et al., 1952a; SCHLESINGER and FRANKEL, 1952a; HAMMON et al., 1960a, b), simian cell cultures (RUSSELL et al., 1966b; YUILL et al., 1968; PAUL, 1968), Aedes aegypti and albopictus mosquitoes via intrathoracic inoculation (McLEAN et al., 1974; ROSEN and GUBLER, 1974), and Aedes albopictus cell cultures (SINGH and PAUL, 1969; CHAPPELL et al., 1971).

2. Mouse

The Swiss albino mouse, first used successfully by KIMURA and HOTTA (1944) and SABIN and SCHLESINGER (1945) for the propagation of dengue-1 virus strains, has remained the experimental animal of choice. The process of "adaptation" of different strains of virus and other aspects of this system will be discussed in appropriate later sections. Suffice it for now to say that, for the production of high-titered stock virus, suckling mice are inoculated with mouse-adapted virus by the intracerebral route. The mice are sacrificed when they show signs of illness (paralysis or other signs referable to pathological involvement of the central nervous system). The brains are harvested and homogenized and serve as the source of virus.

3. Mosquitoes

Although the long-persisting ability of Aedes mosquitoes to transmit dengue virus following an infectious bloodmeal and an extrinsic incubation period had been demonstrated (see Table 2) and carefully documented by SILER et al. (1926), SIMMONS et al. (1931), SABIN (1952a) and others, direct tests for the presence of infectious virus in naturally or experimentally infected mosquitoes became feasible only after the development of assay methods using suckling mice or various cell cultures. Examples of isolation of virus are those reported by HAMMON *et al.* (1960a, b), HALSTEAD *et al.* (1964a), CAREY *et al.* (1964), MYERS *et al.* (1965), RUDNICK and CHAN (1965), RUSSELL *et al.* (1969a, b), and MORALES *et al.* (1973). Replication of mouse-adapted dengue-2 virus after intrathoracic inoculation into *Aedes aegypti* was studied by LAM and MARSHALL (1968), of dengue-1 and -4 by COLEMAN and McLEAN (1973). The same method was used to demonstrate the capacity of *A. aegypti* to transmit human dengue-2 virus to suckling mice (McLEAN *et al.*, 1974) and to develop an infectivity assay for viruses of all four serotypes in *A. albopictus* (ROSEN and GUBLER, 1974; GUBLER and ROSEN, 1976) (see next Section).

4. *In vitro* Cell Cultures

Chick embryo-adapted dengue-1 virus was propagated by SCHLESINGER (1950) through 11 consecutive transfers in tissue minces derived from 5 day-old chick embryos. Propagation of mouse-adapted dengue-1 and -2 viruses in monolayers of trypsin-dispersed rhesus monkey kidney cells was first reported by HOTTA and EVANS (1956a, b). Subsequent workers have shown viral growth in various simian (HALSTEAD *et al.*, 1964b); hamster (DIERCKS and HAMMON, 1958; DIERCKS, 1959; HOTTA *et al.*, 1961; MAGUIRE and MILES, 1965) and the following human cells: conjunctiva and skin (BANTA, 1958; WIEBENGA, 1961a, b), HeLa (BUCKLEY, 1961), KB (BEASLEY *et al.*, 1960; SCHULZE, 1962; SCHULZE and SCHLESINGER, 1963a), miscellaneous (HOTTA *et al.*, 1961). In addition, cell cultures derived from *Aedes aegypti* or *albopictus* have been shown to support replication of dengue viruses (*e.g.*, SINGH and PAUL, 1968, 1969; SUITOR and PAUL, 1969; STEVENS, 1970; CHAPPELL *et al.*, 1971; SINARACHATANANT and OLSON, 1973). Detailed features of these and other systems will be discussed in later sections. In general, virus derived from cell cultures is used in the form of *medium* from infected monolayers.

B. Assay Procedures

1. Infectivity Assays

a) Mice

Mouse-adapted strains of dengue viruses are titrated by intracerebral inoculation of appropriate dilutions of stock virus preparations. Lethal endpoints are estimated by conventional LD_{50} calculations (*e.g.*, REED and MUENCH, 1938).

b) In vitro Cell Cultures

BUCKLEY (1961) described an assay in HeLa cell monolayers under liquid medium based on cytopathic effects (CPE) produced by strains of all four dengue types. This method was later expanded to correlate CPE (CPD_{50}) with LD_{50} in mice, hemagglutinin (HA) production, and hemadsorption (HAd) (BUCKLEY and SRIHONGSE, 1963). For types 1, 2, and 3, especially after many passages in HeLa cell cultures, the titers obtained by these criteria were nearly equivalent. Type 4 gave low titers in cultures. Another assay based on CPE involved KB cells, also an established human line (SCHULZE, 1962; SCHULZE and SCHLESINGER, 1963a). Here again, titers of mouse brain virus in terms of CPD_{50} and LD_{50} were nearly equivalent, provided a properly buffered diluent (in this case, Tris-buffered saline, pH 7.0—7.2, containing gelatin or 0.2% bovine serum albumin) was used.

A *plaque assay* for dengue viruses was introduced by SCHULZE and SCHLESINGER (1963a), utilizing KB cell monolayers and methylcellulose overlay. The latter was substituted for agar because of the exquisite sensitivity to agar polysaccharides of the dengue-1 and -2 strains used (see Section VI. F. on Reaction to Physical and Chemical Agents). Subsequently, hydrolyzed starch or agar mixed with DEAE-dextran were introduced as overlay media and KB cells were replaced by BHK-21 or Vero cells (MILES and AUSTIN, 1963; STOLLAR et al., 1966; BERGOLD and MAZZALI, 1968).

Other workers have introduced plaque assays for different dengue types utilizing the following systems: Rhesus monkey kidney cells (GEORGIADES et al., 1965), monkey kidney cell lines GMK, LLC-MK$_2$, BS-C-1 or Vero (SUKHAVACHANA et al., 1966; HOTTA et al., 1966; BERGOLD and MAZZALI, 1968; STIM, 1969), porcine kidney cells (STIM and HENDERSON, 1966; WESTAWAY, 1966), rabbit kidney cell line MA111 (BERGOLD and MAZZALI, 1968). These various systems have worked in different laboratories with different degrees of success for one or all of the dengue types [cf. the report by BERGOLD and MAZZALI (1968) that BHK-21 cells are suitable for types 1 and 2, not 3 and 4, while AOKI et al. (1967) demonstrated plaque formation by all types tested]. Such "local" variations are to be expected if only because cells, viruses, media, and techniques are never quite the same. Certain variations of the standard plaque assay have utilized "microculture" methods (DE MADRID and PORTERFIELD, 1969, 1974; FUJITA et al., 1975). Others have proved especially useful for qualitative work and for initial isolation and identification of field strains (YUILL et al., 1968).

Much of the work to be described in the sections dealing with the physical-chemical characterization of dengue-2 virions was based on the plaque assay initially developed by SCHULZE and SCHLESINGER (1963a), the current modification of which involves BHK-21, LLC-MK$_2$, or Vero cells. The same basic technique, utilizing KB cells, has been used successfully for plaque assays of all types of dengue virus (SCHLESINGER and STEVENS, unpublished). The need for DEAE-dextran or for methylcellulose or hydrolyzed starch as substitutes for agar is, of course, dependent on the extent to which any given virus strain is inhibited by sulfated agar polysaccharides (SCHULZE and SCHLESINGER, 1963b; SCHULZE, 1964). This can be easily ascertained by HA titration in presence of aqueous agar extracts (see Section VI. F.). It should be emphasized that BHK-21 cells, like many other established cell lines, are heterogenous and subject to karyotypic variation (DEFENDI et al., 1963). This may be reflected in variations in the ability of different cloned sublines to support plaque formation by dengue viruses.

A method currently in routine use employs Vero cells. Confluent monolayers in plastic Petri plates are washed with phosphate-buffered saline (PBS) and then inoculated with appropriate dilutions of virus. The diluent is Tris-buffered saline containing 0.4% bovine serum albumin, pH 8 (BAT). After an adsorption period of 90 minutes at 37° C, the inoculum is removed, and the cell layer is overlaid with 9 ml of Eagle's basic medium (BME, EAGLE, 1955) containing double-strength amino acids and vitamins, 10% horse serum, 0.15% tryptose phosphate, 500 µg/ml DEAE-dextran, and 0.9% agar. Cultures are incubated at 37° C in a 5% CO$_2$-air atmosphere. After 4 days, neutral red is added. Plaques are clearly visible after a few hours at 37° C and remain so for 3—4 days. Detailed studies of several variables influencing efficiency of plaque formation have been reported by STIM (1970a, b).

Finally, fluorescent focus assays have been reported for clone isolation of certain strains of dengue-2 (LUBINIECKI et al., 1973) and for rapid infectivity titrations of dengue-4 virus (IGARASHI and MANTANI, 1974).

c) Mosquitoes

ROSEN and GUBLER (1974) reported that virus titration by intrathoracic inoculation into female or male A. albopictus is equivalent or superior in sensitivity to intracerebral titration in suckling mice or plaque titrations on LLC-MK$_2$ cell cultures. In their work they used the latter method to assay virus titers attained in the whole triturated individual mosquito. The utility of the mosquito assay procedure was demonstrated for strains of all four serotypes in the form of either human sera, mouse-adapted, or LLC-MK$_2$ cell-derived virus.

2. Hemagglutination

The capacity of dengue viruses to agglutinate chick red blood cells (RBC) was initially demonstrated by SWEET and SABIN (1954). These authors were the first to describe the apparent paradox exhibited by dengue-1 and -2 viruses, in common with other group B togaviruses, with regard to optimal pH required for stability of the HA capacity on one hand (7.9 or higher) and for the HA reaction itself on the other (6.2—6.9). Their basic observations were confirmed and extended to a large number of other group A and B togaviruses by CASALS and BROWN (1954) and CLARKE and CASALS (1958). NAKAGAWA and SHINGU (1955) and SHINGU (1955, 1956) introduced horse RBC and reported on the function of Ca^{++} ions in stabilizing the HA property of the virus as well as the HA reaction itself. PORTERFIELD (1957) recommended the use of goose RBC, and finally CLARKE and CASALS (1958) synthesized all available knowledge in a comprehensive survey of optimal conditions for HA by many different arboviruses.

For dengue viruses, the following method is recommended: *(a) Preparation and storage of viral HA:* depending on source material (see section on Purification); *(b) Diluent for viral HA:* BABS 9, *i.e.,* crystalline bovine serum albumin, 0.2%, in borate-saline, pH 9 (H$_3$BO$_3$ 0.05 M, NaCl 0.12 M, adjusted to pH 9 with 24 ml of 1 M NaOH per liter); *(c) Goose RBC:* mix fresh citrated goose blood with 2.5—3 vol. of DGV (dextrose-gelatin-veronal) buffer; wash 4× in same vol. of DGV; resuspend final RBC pellet in DGV and adjust to desired stock density (about 8% v/v); stock suspension is stable at 2—4° C for at least 3 weeks; *(d) for test:* make 2-fold serial dilutions of viral HA in BABS 9 (volume depending on type of tray or tubes used); dilute stock suspension of RBC 1:40 (to O.D.$_{490}$ = 0.450 or to about 0.2% v/v) in 0.15 M NaCl—0.2 M phosphate buffer of such composition that final reaction mixture after addition to equal volume of viral HA dilutions will have desired pH (6.2—6.9). The RBC suspension should be kept in an ice bath. The HA reaction itself can be incubated in the cold or at room temperature. Positive, negative, and intermediate reactions are read as in the pattern test for influenza virus originally described by SALK (1944).

For further technical details, the paper by CLARKE and CASALS (1958) should be consulted. More precise directions concerning final pH and temperature are not given here because experience in several laboratories has taught that, within the limits given, optimal conditions have to be worked out for each strain and source material.

In general, the association of dengue viral HA with goose erythrocytes is stable (STEVENS and SCHLESINGER, 1965). The claim by NAKAGAWA and SHINGU (1957) that elution of virus adsorbed on horse RBC can be achieved by reduction of divalent cation concentration is not convincingly borne out by their data.

C. Serological Procedures

1. Neutralization

a) In Mice

The neutralization test originally developed by SABIN and SCHLESINGER (described by SABIN, 1948b) was patterned after the method still used by some workers for arboviruses in general:

A constant concentration (usually undiluted) of test serum is mixed with serial dilutions of stock virus; the mixture is incubated for 2 hours at 37° C; aliquots of each mixture are inoculated intracerebrally into mice; neutralization is read in terms of survival of mice, i.e., as the difference of virus titer in presence and in absence of the test serum; the $\log_{10}$ of this difference is called the neutralization index (NI); a value of < 1.0 is interpreted as negative, 1.0—1.7 as equivocal, > 1.7 as positive. A modification introduced by SABIN (1950) was based on the observation that a maximal NI was obtained only when (a) fresh or frozen immune serum was used or (b) the inactivating effect of heating the serum at 56° for 30 min. was compensated for by adding to the reaction mixture fresh or frozen normal serum ("heat-labile accessory factor"). The functions or nature of this factor are not clearly understood, and several subsequent reports (e.g., SCHLESINGER et al., 1956; HAMMON et al., 1966; BANERJEE, 1967) have described equivalent NI values for tests with native and heat-inactivated sera in the presence or absence of fresh normal serum.

Recent studies by STOLLAR (1975) have revealed that complement does enhance neutralization of purified Sindbis virus (an alphavirus) by heated antiviral serum and that this enhancement is associated with complement-dependent injury to the viral envelope (as measured by accessibility of radioactively labeled nucleocapsid RNA to ribonuclease, with consequent release of TCA soluble radioactivity). This effect is, however, seen only at optimal serum dilutions with distinct inactive prozone at high concentrations. Such a mechanism may explain the inconsistencies of complement enhancement observed in standard neutralization tests with dengue and other togaviruses.

Of more crucial importance is the question of the validity of the NI as a reliable quantitative measure of antibody activity or, indeed, as a test of *specific* neutralization. This question has been discussed on theoretical grounds by FAZEKAS DE ST. GROTH (1962) who concludes: "It follows that the titer of an antiserum can be determined much more accurately by using the constant virus, variable serum arrangement . . . than by its opposite (constant serum, variable virus . . .). The latter is only justified as a measure of despair, when no reaction can be obtained except with undiluted antiserum. Even here it would seem much sounder to explore some of the means by which sensitivity can be enhanced before giving in and accepting a technique that is uninformative, wasteful of material, and prone to nonspecific inhibition". These drawbacks apply regardless of whether the test with undiluted serum is evaluated as stated (death vs. survival) or with the refinement of considering average survival time (SMITH and WESTGARTH, 1957).

WISSEMAN *et al*. (1966) sought to quantitate the intracerebral neutralization test by using the serum dilution/fixed virus dose (10—100 LD_{50}) method. As has been the experience of other workers, certain sera which gave respectable NI's when tested undiluted yielded titers of less than 1:2 when examined in the more quantitative test. Regardless of which method is used, the key difficulty of the intracerebral test resides in the fact that the scoring criterion is an all-or-none effect, and that any infectious particles escaping neutralization can theoretically initiate the events that bring about the death of an experimental animal. Hence effective neutralization will require a huge excess of antibody and specificity is not assured. It is for these reasons that greater reliability and specificity are provided by quantitative neutralization assays in which the scoring criterion is the effective inactivation of single viral particles (plaque neutralization).

b) Plaque Reduction

The development of a plaque assay for dengue viruses (SCHULZE, 1962; SCHULZE and SCHLESINGER, 1963a) permitted the quantitation of antibodies by the plaque reduction technique (SCHULZE, 1962). RUSSELL *et al*. (1967) subjected their plaque reduction test on LLC-MK₂ cells to careful probit analysis and established the high degree of specificity (RUSSELL and NISALAK, 1967) and accuracy of antibody titers measured in this way.

Further applications and comparisons of these and related methods in studies on strain and type differentiation and identification will be discussed in later sections.

2. Hemagglutination Inhibition (HI)

The principles of the HI test employ those of the HA reaction already discussed. The crucial requirement is the removal from test sera of non-specific inhibitors (probably lipids or lipoproteins) and of agglutinins present in many normal sera. For the former, SWEET and SABIN (1954a) and CASALS and BROWN (1954) originally recommended the use of acetone extraction. Their procedure has been replaced, for routine purposes, by the empirical kaolin adsorption method of CLARKE and CASALS (1958).

Twenty-five grams of acid-washed kaolin powder are suspended in 100 ml of borate saline, pH 9.0 (BS 9). Heat-inactivated (56° for 30 min.) serum, diluted ¹/₅ with BS 9, is mixed with an equal volume of 25% kaolin, kept at room temperature for 20 min. with occasional agitation, and centrifuged at 2500 rpm for 10 min. The resulting supernatant is then considered as ¹/₁₀ serum. This is subjected to adsorption with a goose RBC suspension in the cold to remove normal agglutinins. To 2-fold serial dilutions of the final product in BS 9 are added equal volumes of HA antigen representing 4—8 HA units per well or tube (also diluted in BS 9). The mixtures are incubated overnight at 2—4° C, then the RBC are added and the tests incubated and read as described above under HA. The extent of cross reactions encountered in this type of test will be discussed under Antigenic Structure (Section VI. E.).

3. Complement Fixation (CF)

SABIN and YOUNG (1949) first reported the detection of CF antigen in aqueous extracts of dengue-1 infected suckling mouse brains. This antigen cross-reacted with sera of human dengue-2 convalescent sera at lower titers than those in the homologous system (SABIN and YOUNG, 1949; SABIN, 1950). The converse relationship was demonstrated for similarly prepared dengue-2 antigens after a representative strain had been adapted to mice (SCHLESINGER and FRANKEL, 1952a). Subsequent work by CASALS and his coworkers established the extent of cross reactivity of dengue antigens with other group B togaviruses (see Section VI. E. on Antigenic Structure).

4. Immunodiffusion

Standard procedures for agar gel diffusion (CHAN, 1965; HAWKES and MARSHALL, 1967; IBRAHIM and HAMMON, 1968a) and immunoelectrophoresis (CUADRADO and CASALS, 1967; IBRAHIM and HAMMON, 1968b) have been applied to antigenic analyses of dengue viruses. The results will be discussed under Antigenic Structure (Section VI. E.).

VI. Properties of the Dengue Virion

A. Size and Morphology

1. Filtration

The initial filtration experiments by ASHBURN and CRAIG (1907) and CLELAND et al. (1919) were refined by MANOUSSAKIS (1928) who found that dengue virus, in the form of infectious human serum, could pass Chamberland L II filters, indicating a relatively small size of the viral particles. Later estimates of the particle diameter determined by the gradocol membrane technique and infectivity of the filtrate for human volunteers were reported as 13—23 nm by TODA and NAKAGAWA (1943, 1944) and 17—25 nm or less by SABIN (1952a). More recent electron microscopic evidence indicates that these values are too low, at least for the enveloped, complete virions. One may suggest three alternative explanations of this apparent discrepancy: (a) defects of the filters or the filtration procedures or their interpretation, (b) distortion of the enveloped virions during filtration, (c) infectiousness of naked viral cores for experimental human subjects. Passage of infectious mouse-adapted dengue-2 virions through Millipore filters of 50 nm average pore diameter has been reported by CASALS (1968b).

2. Electron Microscopy

In early phases of electron microscopic studies, several different kinds of structures were observed. In 1945, SABIN, SCHLESINGER, and STANLEY (reported in SABIN, 1952a) examined pelleted material from differentially centrifuged, highly infectious, human serum. They found dumbell-shaped structures measuring 700×20—40 nm which were not found in similarly prepared sediments of normal human sera. Different, rod-like structures (175—200×42—46 nm) were found by REAGAN and BRUECKNER (1952a) in the pellets of dengue-infected mouse brain homogenates subjected to centrifugation at 44,770 rpm for 3 hours. The possible significance of these findings cannot be evaluated.

OZAWA (1954) described spherical bodies, 34.2 ± 2.8 nm in diameter, in infected mouse brain homogenates centrifuged at 30,000 rpm for one hour. His preparations, however, apparently did not lose infectivity after treatment with ethyl ether, a result not consistent with the ether sensitivity of dengue virus.

Of probably greater interest are small particles found in infected mouse brain homogenates by HOTTA (1953a). The virus (dengue-1, Mochizuki strain) was partially purified by a kaolin absorption method. Spherical bodies, approximately 20 nm in diameter, were noted which were not found in control non-infected mouse brain homogenates.

NAKAGAWA and SHINGU (1957) examined dengue-1 virus (Hawaiian strain) grown either in mouse brain or in chick embryos. They purified the materials by adsorption and elution on horse erythrocytes or by protamine sulfate precipitation, both combined with ultracentrifugation at $90,000 \times g$ for 60 minutes. In such specimens, round particles, 18 ± 2 nm in diameter, were revealed, which showed a tendency to aggregate.

In light of more recent observations of intact or degraded virions and of virus-infected cells, it seems possible that these particles may have represented viral cores either in the form of cell-associated precursors or of virions stripped of their envelopes.

For example, MATSUMURA and HOTTA (1967; 1971) purified mouse-passaged type 1 virus by a method combining protamine precipitation, zonal centrifugation and sucrose density gradient centrifugation. In fractions showing dengue-specific hemagglutinating activity, negative staining with phosphotungstic acid (PTA) revealed spherical particles, 50—60 nm in diameter, with projections around the "envelope". Additionally, small particles, about 20—30 nm in diameter, and pleomorphic structures such as larger forms and "empty" particles apparently lacking an inner "core" were also noted. No structures similar to these were observed in control materials obtained from uninfected mouse brains.

More homogeneous round structures were seen in "rapidly sedimenting HA" (RHA) fractions isolated from sucrose gradients of dengue-2 virus isolated from infected mouse brain by SMITH et al. (1970). The RHA fraction corresponded to peak infectivity and can therefore be assumed to represent infectious virions (see Section VI. B. 3.). The particles, negatively stained with uranyl acetate, were 48—50 nm in diameter and showed a mottled surface structure in which ring-shaped "subunits" of 7 nm diameter with a 1—2 nm "hole" could be discerned. "Subunits" of this type were also found to separate from disintegrating virions after several days' storage at 4° C. An additional structure, a "doughnut" 14 nm in diameter with a negatively stained 5 to 7 nm central zone, was characteristic of the SHA ("slowly sedimenting HA" fraction) (see Section VI. B. 3.).

MATSUMURA et al. (1971) examined partially purified dengue-2 virions obtained from infected KB cell cultures. The particles appeared uniform in size and round, with an average diameter of 48—50 nm (Fig. 5a). At higher magnification, they showed a central portion, 40 nm in diameter, external to which there was an unstained zone of about 30 Å width, and then an outer layer projecting to a width of about 2 nm (Figs. 5b, c). Further details of the virion structure were not resolved by negative staining. Osmotic shock of dengue-2 virions (by exposure to 4.0 M NaCl) led to the appearance of structures measuring about 26 nm along with "empty shells". It was suggested (MATSUMURA *et al.*, 1971) that the 26 nm structures might represent viral nucleocapsids or cores and that the "empty shells" might be either envelopes or, alternately, perhaps distorted forms of the cores.

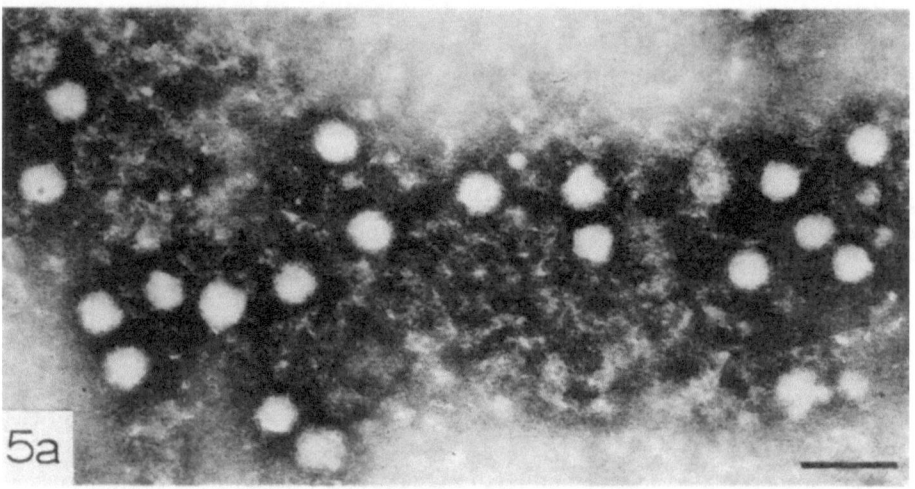

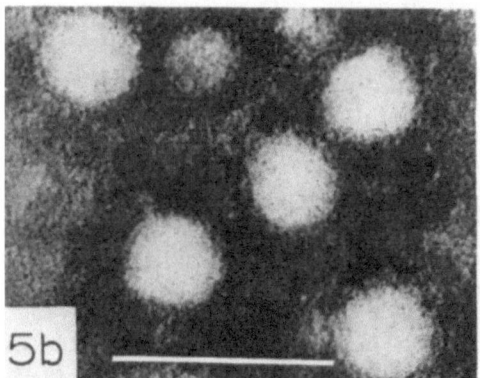
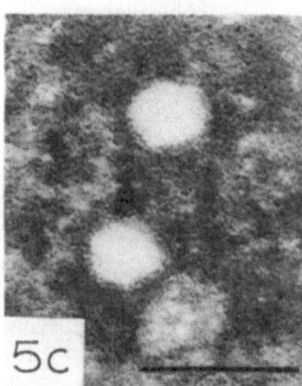

Fig. 5. Electron micrographs of partially purified dengue-2 virions, negatively stained with phosphotungstic acid.
Bars represent 100 nm. (a) demonstrates relatively homogenous shape and diameter; (b) and (c) show a fringe of projections, with their periodicity especially evident on the lower particle in (c). Modified from MATSUMURA *et al.*, 1971

DEMSEY *et al.* (1974) have employed the freeze-fracture technique in an attempt to resolve virion structure in greater detail. Of perhaps greatest interest is their interpretation of preferred fracture lines as indicating that the viral envelope is almost entirely a lipid bilayer, lacking the proteins usually observed in cell membrane-associated particles. The projections measuring 7 nm are removed by one of the fractures, leaving a smooth membrane structure.

Neither these studies nor those on dengue-1 virions by MATSUMURA and HOTTA (1971) have succeeded in clarifying the basic structure and symmetry of the viral nucleocapsid.

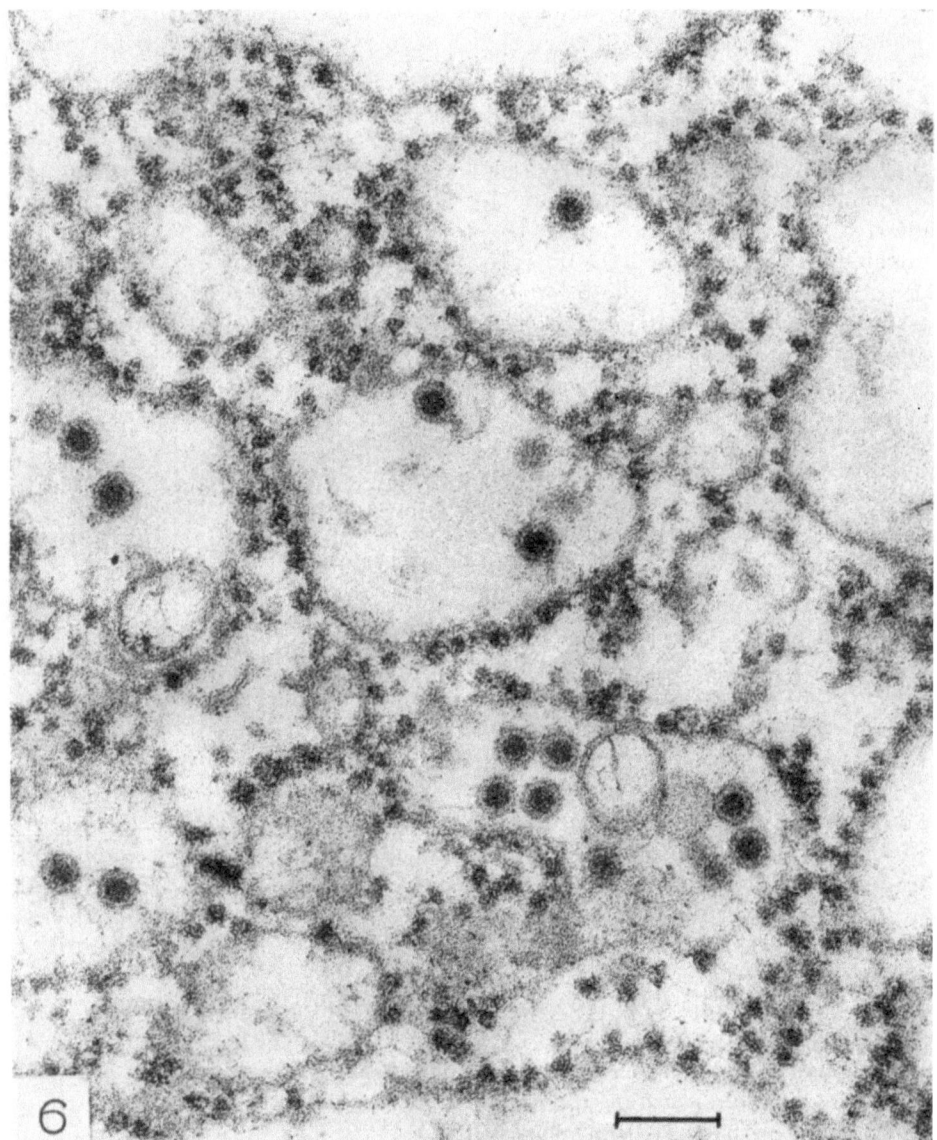

Fig. 6. Thin section of Vero cell, 24 hours after infection with dengue-2 virus (m.o.i. 30 PFU/cell).
Virions showing 26 nm electron dense core, separated from a "knobby" envelope by a lucent zone of approx. 4 nm width. Virions are located in vesicles studded on the cytoplasmic side with electron dense bodies. It is not known whether these are viral nucleocapsids or ribosomes (see also Figs. 18, 19, 21). Bar = 100 nm. Modified from MATSUMURA *et al.*, 1971

Additional insight into the structure, development, and release of dengue virions has been derived from electron microscopic study of thin sections of infected cells. OHYAMA *et al.* (1967), employing Epon embedding and uranium acetate-lead acetate double staining, prepared thin sections of mouse brains and an established line of green monkey kidney cells, both infected with type 4 virus originating from patients with Thai hemorrhagic fever; in either kind of specimens were found spherical particles of 40—50 nm in diameter, having an electron-dense "core" approximately 20 nm in diameter. In the early stage of infection the particles were apparently situated within the cells, and in the later stages they appeared also extracellularly. Some of them were shown to aggregate.

Similar observations were made by MATSUMURA *et al.* (1971) on dengue-2 infected Vero cells. The example illustrated in Fig. 6 shows the knobby membrane of the viral envelope, and the cross-section of the electron-dense core. Although it would be nice to conclude from the latter feature that the nucleocapsid of the virion has cubic symmetry (cf. HORZINEK, 1973a, b), this would be premature in absence of any discernible subunit arrangement. Further discussions of thin section and freeze-fracture electron microscopy will be found in Section VII (Viral Replication).

B. Purification

1. Preliminary Extraction or Precipitation of Virus-Containing Materials

Techniques reported to be utilizable for the partial purification of dengue viruses include: kaolin adsorption (HOTTA, 1953a); protamine sulfate treatment (NAKAGAWA, 1953); DEAE cellulose column chromatography (TAKEHARA and HOTTA, 1961; SMITH *et al.*, 1970); fluorocarbon treatment (TAKEHARA and HOTTA, 1961; STEVENS and SCHLESINGER, 1965); combined treatment with protamine sulfate and ethanol. The latter method was applied by MATSUMURA *et al.* (1967) to the partial purification of dengue-1 virus in the form of infected mouse brain homogenates. Protamine sulfate, 1 mg/ml, was added to crude stock virus. The precipitate formed after 1 hour was centrifuged at low speed. To the supernatant fraction was added 25% (v/v) prechilled ethanol. The mixture was held at 4° C for 60 minutes with occasional shaking. Most of the activity (LD_{50} and HA) was recovered in the ethanol precipitate resuspended in Tris-cystine-saline (0.14 M NaCl in Tris buffer containing 0.1 M cystine, pH 8.0). The purification achieved was about 50-fold in terms of LD_{50} per mg protein, about 250-fold in terms of HA units per mg protein.

Additional methods of partial purification employ precipitation with 50% (STEVENS and SCHLESINGER, 1963) or 30—70% (STOLLAR, 1969) saturated ammonium sulfate with subsequent resuspension in BABS 9 or adsorption on aluminum phosphate gel (MILLER and SCHLESINGER, 1955) followed by elution into pH 9 buffer containing 0.5—1.0 M NaCl (STEVENS and SCHLESINGER, 1963).

Selective adsorption of ^{32}P-labeled dengue-2 virus on goose RBC was used by STEVENS and SCHLESINGER (1965) to monitor relative distribution of radioactivity incorporated into viral populations with different biological properties (see below). These authors were unable to elute dengue-2 virus from RBC, but NAKAGAWA and SHINGU (1957) have reported success in eluting dengue-1 virus from horse RBC as a step in their purification procedure.

2. Preparative Centrifugation

STEVENS and SCHLESINGER (1965) compared the effectiveness of direct pelleting and of centrifugation of virus onto a cushion of fluorocarbon (density at 25° = 1.574 g/ml). Initially, the recovery of infectious virus [in terms of plaque-forming units (PFU)] was more quantitative and more reproducible by the second method. More recently, however, it has seemed preferable to avoid use of fluorocarbon. Accordingly, virus-containing medium from infected cell cultures has been subjected to preliminary low speed centrifugation, with or without intervening $(NH_4)_2SO_4$ precipitation, followed by direct pelleting at $78,000 \times g$ for 2 hours at 4° C (STOLLAR et al., 1966; STOLLAR, 1969). When the resulting pellet is resuspended in $1/50$ to $1/100$ the original volume of BABS 9, followed by homogenization in a Dounce microhomogenizer, quantitative recovery in terms of PFU and HAU is readily achieved.

3. Gradient Centrifugation

It has been a consistent finding that populations of dengue-2 or dengue-1 viral particles, partially purified by any of the preparative steps outlined above, are heterogeneous with regard to buoyant density, sedimentation velocity, relative infectiousness, and chemical composition. It was first shown by STEVENS and SCHLESINGER (1963, 1965) that dengue-2 virus derived from infected KB cell cultures and subjected to CsCl equilibrium density gradient centrifugation yielded two major HA components with mean densities of 1.24 and 1.19 g/ml, respectively. 95—99% of the infectivity (PFU) was associated with the heavier component, with disproportionately high infectivity toward the densest region (Fig. 7a). When fractions from each of the two major HA bands were combined (pool I and II in Fig. 7b) and subjected to a second CsCl density gradient centrifugation, clean separation was achieved. As shown in Figure 7b, the denser band sometimes resolved itself into two subcomponents. A similar distribution of HA density bands was found by MATSUMURA et al. (1967) for dengue-1 virus and by SMITH et al. (1970) for dengue-2 virus, both derived from mouse brain. The latter authors, while confirming the density peaks of HA components derived from cell cultures as 1.24 and 1.19 g/ml, observed that mouse brain virus was shifted to 1.22 and 1.18 g/ml, suggesting different lipid contents. That the HA activity associated with both components was indeed virus-specific was demonstrated by STEVENS and SCHLESINGER (1965) who found that the attachment to goose RBC of ^{32}P-labeled "complete" and "incomplete" virus from CsCl gradients was inhibited to comparable extent by pretreatment with dengue-2 specific antiserum.

Proper interpretation of these findings is compromised by the marked loss of infectivity (>100-fold in 48 hours) of dengue-2 virus in presence of CsCl at the concentration used in the gradient runs (STEVENS and SCHLESINGER, 1965). Replacement of CsCl by Cs_2SO_4, potassium tartrate, or sucrose equilibrium density gradients did not consistently eliminate this difficulty (STEVENS, unpublished observations).

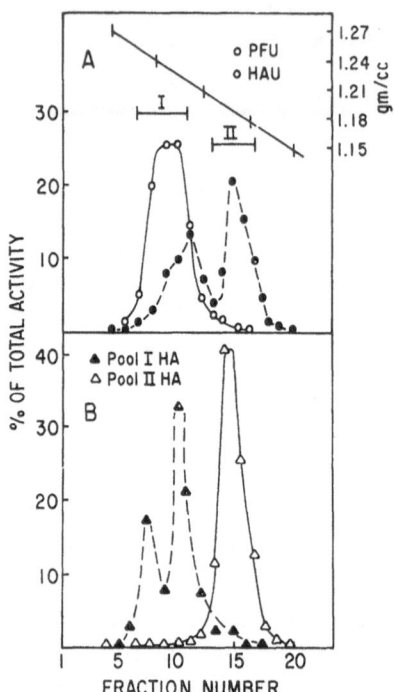

Fig. 7. Two consecutive CsCl density gradient centrifugations of partially purified dengue-2 virus.
The activity of each fraction is expressed as the percentage of the total activity recovered in all fractions. Panel (A) depicts infectivity and HA activity of each fraction after the first run, Panel (B) HA activity after recentrifugation of Pool I and II fractions indicated in Panel (A). Modified from STEVENS and SCHLESINGER, 1965

Rate zonal centrifugation in 5—25% sucrose gradients for 3 hours at 25,000 rpm also resulted in separation of two major HA components (STOLLAR et al., 1966; SMITH et al., 1970). Again, more than 95% of the plaque-forming activity was associated with the more rapidly sedimenting component (Fig. 8) and a total of 30 to 100% of the original PFU were recovered (STOLLAR et al., 1966). A similar, but somewhat more heterodisperse pattern was found by MATSUMURA et al. (1967) for mouse brain-derived dengue-1 virus. It should be noted that the heterogeneity of dengue-2 virus was observed under conditions which yielded a single sharp band of Sindbis virus (STOLLAR, 1969). Because the physical differences between the more rapidly and the more slowly sedimenting particles were well correlated with their distinguishing biological and chemical features, they were referred to as "complete" and "incomplete" virus, respectively. SMITH et al. (1970) reported that their corresponding sucrose gradient peaks ("RHA" and "SHA") reacted in HI tests to the same degree with antiviral antibodies.

According to ROSATO et al. (1974) and WESTAWAY et al. (1975), the sedimentation coefficient of dengue virions ("RHA"), as determined in 15—30% sucrose velocity gradients, is 200S (compared with 240S for Sindbis virions), that of "SHA" 70 to 85S.

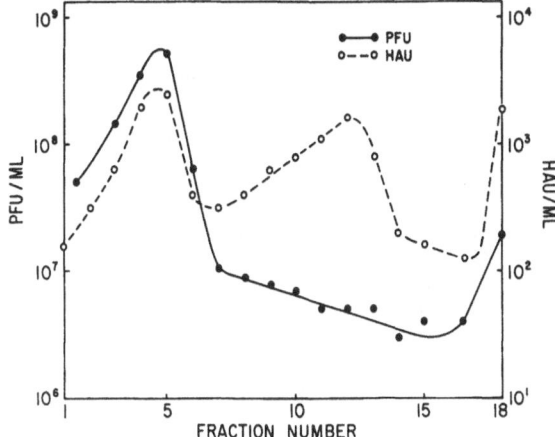

Fig. 8. Infectivity and hemagglutinin titers of virus fractions from a sucrose gradient. Two milliliters of virus concentrate was layered on a 27-ml linear sucrose gradient (5—25%) and centrifuged for 3 hours at 25,000 rpm in the Spinco SW 25.1 rotor. (Fractions 1—2 and 16—17 were pooled for plaque titrations.) Centrifugation from right to left. From STOLLAR *et al.* (1966)
With permission of the authors and Academic Press, Inc., New York

C. Chemical Composition

Like other group A and B togaviruses that have been chemically analyzed (cf. PFEFFERKORN, 1968; PFEFFERKORN and SHAPIRO, 1974), dengue viruses contain RNA, lipids, proteins, and carbohydrates. The RNA nature of dengue viral genetic material was initially inferred from the fact that phenol extraction of infected mouse brain yielded an infectious ribonuclease-sensitive principle (ADA and ANDERSON, 1959; NAKAMURA, 1961; SCHULZE, 1962).

1. Lipids

The presence of lipids was indicated initially by the sensitivity of different viral strains to ethyl ether (HOTTA and EVANS, 1956 c), deoxycholate (THEILER, 1957), and pancreatic lipase (TAKEHARA and HOTTA, 1961). Direct evidence for the presence of lipids stems from fractionation of ^{32}P-labeled dengue-2 virus (STEVENS and SCHLESINGER, 1965). In these experiments, the labeled virus was adsorbed selectively to goose RBC, and the latter served at the same time as a convenient source of non-radioactive carrier macromolecules. When ^{32}P-labeled, complete and incomplete viral populations from CsCl density gradients were analyzed in this way, the amount of label incorporated into the lipid fractions proved to be constant relative to the HA titer. In contrast, the amount of label incorporated into RNA was directly proportional to infectious titers, not to HA titers (see next Section). By analogy to group A togaviruses (cf. PFEFFERKORN and SHAPIRO, 1974), one would expect the lipid composition of dengue virions to reflect that of the host cell from which they are derived and to vary accordingly. No such data are available.

2. Viral RNA

STOLLAR *et al.* (1966) studied the characteristics of RNA extracted with phenol at room temperature from "complete" and "incomplete" dengue-2 virus (sucrose gradient fractions). The complete virus yielded a major species of RNA with a sedimentation coefficient estimated at 45S. As shown in Fig. 9. this RNA is

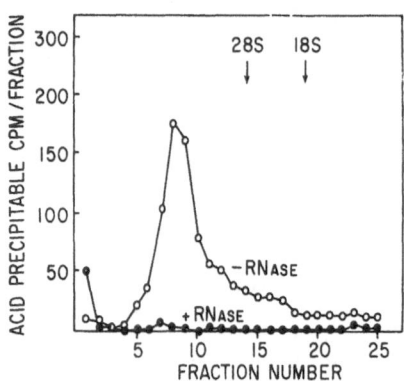

Fig. 9. Ribonuclease sensitivity of 45S RNA isolated from ^{3}H-uridine labeled dengue-2 virus ("RHA" fraction of a sucrose gradient).
A mixture of labeled RNA and unlabeled rat liver RNA in a total volume of 1.0 ml was layered on 28 ml of a sucrose gradient (5—20%) which was run at 21,000 rpm for 16 ½ hours in the SW 25.1 rotor. One milliliter fractions were collected and O.D.$_{260}$ on each was determined. Each fraction was then divided into two equal parts. The acid-precipitable counts were measured directly on one part and after treatment with RNase (final concentration 1 µg/ml in 0.15 M NaCl at 37° for 20 minutes), on the other part.
Modified from STOLLAR *et al.* (1966)

completely degraded by ribonuclease. It is rich in purine base (Table 4), with adenine as the main component. For comparison, Table 5 shows base ratios of other togaviruses which are similar with regard to the relatively high adenine content. Sensitivity to ribonuclease and lack of base pairing indicate that the 45S RNA is single-stranded.

A small amount of 45S RNA of the same characteristics is also associated with the "incomplete" virus obtained from sucrose gradients (Table 4). As shown in Table 6, the amount of label incorporated into the 45S RNA of both, ,,complete" (RHA) and "incomplete" (SHA), viral bands is proportional to the number of virions registering as PFU. Hence, the 45S RNA associated with "incomplete" virus represents the trailing portion of complete, infectious particles (1—3% of the total PFU).

Of perhaps greater interest is the finding that the "incomplete" (SHA) virus contains, in addition, a significant amount of 6—8S RNA (Fig. 10) the base composition of which differs from that of the 45S species (Table 4). The nature and origin of this RNA have not yet been clarified.

STOLLAR *et al.* (1966) estimated a molecular weight of 3.3×10^6 for the 45S dengue-2 viral RNA, calculated according to AGRAWAL and BRUENING (1966).

Table 4. *Base ratios of RNA's from "complete" and "incomplete" dengue-2 particles*

Gradient fraction	RNA fraction	Moles per 100 moles of base			
		A	U	G	C
"RHA"	45S	30.6	21.6	26.4	21.3
"SHA"	45S	31.3	21.8	25.2	21.8
"SHA"	6—8S	24.4	24.4	29.1	22.1

Modified from STOLLAR *et al.* (1966).

Table 5. *Base ratios of the virion RNA of various togaviruses*

Virus	Group	Moles per 100 moles of base				Reference
		Ade-nine	Ura-cil	Gua-nine	Cyto-sine	
Sindbis	A	29.6	19.7	25.8	24.9	PFEFFERKORN AND HUNTER (1963a)
Semliki Forest	A	27.4	22.2	26.1	24.4	SONNABEND *et al.* (1967)
Semliki Forest	A	29.4	19.5	25.5	25.9	KÄÄRIÄINEN and GOMATOS (1969)
Western equine encephalitis	A	29.6	22.7	22.3	25.3	SREEVALSAN *et al.* (1968)
Chikungunya	A	32.9	23.5	21.3	22.2	NAGATOMO (1972)
Murray Valley encephalitis	B	25.5	25.5	27.5	21.5	ADA *et al.* (1962)
St. Louis encephalitis	B	30.7	21.4	26.2	21.7	TRENT *et al.* (1969)

Modified from PFEFFERKORN and SHAPIRO (1974).

Table 6. *Radioactivity of 45S RNA from "RHA" and "SHA" fractions in relation to infectivity prior to extraction*

Exp.	Gradient fraction	PFU/ml	Cpm/ml[a]	Cpm/PFU
1	RHA	2.6×10^8	8.05×10^4	3.1×10^{-4}
	SHA	6.9×10^6	1.85×10^{3b}	2.7×10^{-4}
2	RHA	5.6×10^8	4.6×10^4	0.82×10^{-4}
	SHA	1.2×10^7	2.2×10^{3b}	1.8×10^{-4}
3	RHA	2.3×10^9	1.65×10^5	7.2×10^{-5}
	SHA	3.8×10^7	3.5×10^{3b}	9.2×10^{-5}

[a] Trichloroacetic acid precipitable counts. All three experiments were done with ^{32}P-labeled virus.

[b] In the case of RNA from SHA fractions, the proportion in the 45S fraction was estimated by sucrose gradient analysis. The figures above represent only the 45S species of RNA.

Modified from STOLLAR *et al.* (1966).

This value was initially questioned by PFEFFERKORN (1968) on the basis of the subsequent report by STOLLAR et al. (1967) of the characteristics of the 20 S replicative form of dengue-2 viral RNA (see Section VII on Viral Replication). PFEFFERKORN suggested that "since the hydrodynamic properties of double-stranded RNA's are probably quite uniform, this . . . may indicate that the arboviruses contain an RNA molecule of the molecular weight established for picornavirus RNA, i.e., about 2×10^6". On the other hand, SIMMONS and STRAUSS (1972), using centrifugation in dimethyl sulfoxide (DMSO), calculated a sedimentation coefficient of 49 S for the RNA of Sindbis virus (42 S by other methods) to which they assigned a MW of 4.3×10^6 daltons.

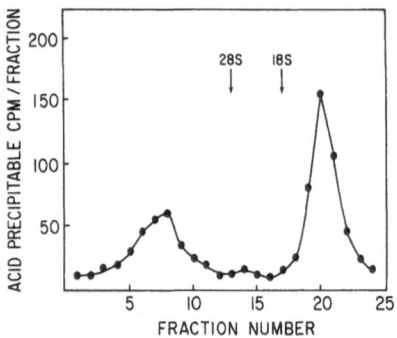

Fig. 10. Sucrose gradient analysis of ^{32}P-labeled RNA from the "SHA" fraction of dengue-2 virus.
Viral RNA and rat liver RNA (total volume 0.25 ml) were layered on a 4.8 ml sucrose gradient and centrifuged at 39,000 rpm for $3\frac{1}{2}$ hours in the SW 39 rotor. Fractions were collected, and each was diluted with 1.00 ml of H_2O. Modified from STOLLAR et al. (1966)

Workers at the Walter Reed Army Institute of Research (P. K. RUSSELL, personal communication) have subjected RNA's from purified EEE, WEE, Japanese encephalitis, and dengue-2 virus to co-electrophoresis on polyacrylamide gels with Sindbis RNA and found them all to move at comparable rates. Use of chick cell ribosomal RNA as marker indicated a molecular weight in the range of 3.7—4.2×10^6 daltons, with a mean of 3.9×10^6 daltons, for all of them. Similarly BOULTON and WESTAWAY (1972) determined an average molecular weight of 4.2×10^6 daltons for both Sindbis (group A) and Kunjin (group B) viruses. This value is accepted as the best current estimate for dengue viral RNA.

Information about the structure of the virion RNA molecule is lacking. Circumstantial evidence suggesting that it is of "plus", i.e. messenger, polarity consists of its infectiousness and mode of replication (Sections VI. D. 1. and VII. C.). The presence of polyadenylate sequences associated with the genome has not been demonstrated.

3. Viral Structural Proteins

The separation of dengue-2 viral populations by rate zonal centrifugation in sucrose gradients into "complete" (RHA) and "incomplete" (SHA) HA particles is again reflected in the distribution of label incorporated into virus grown in KB

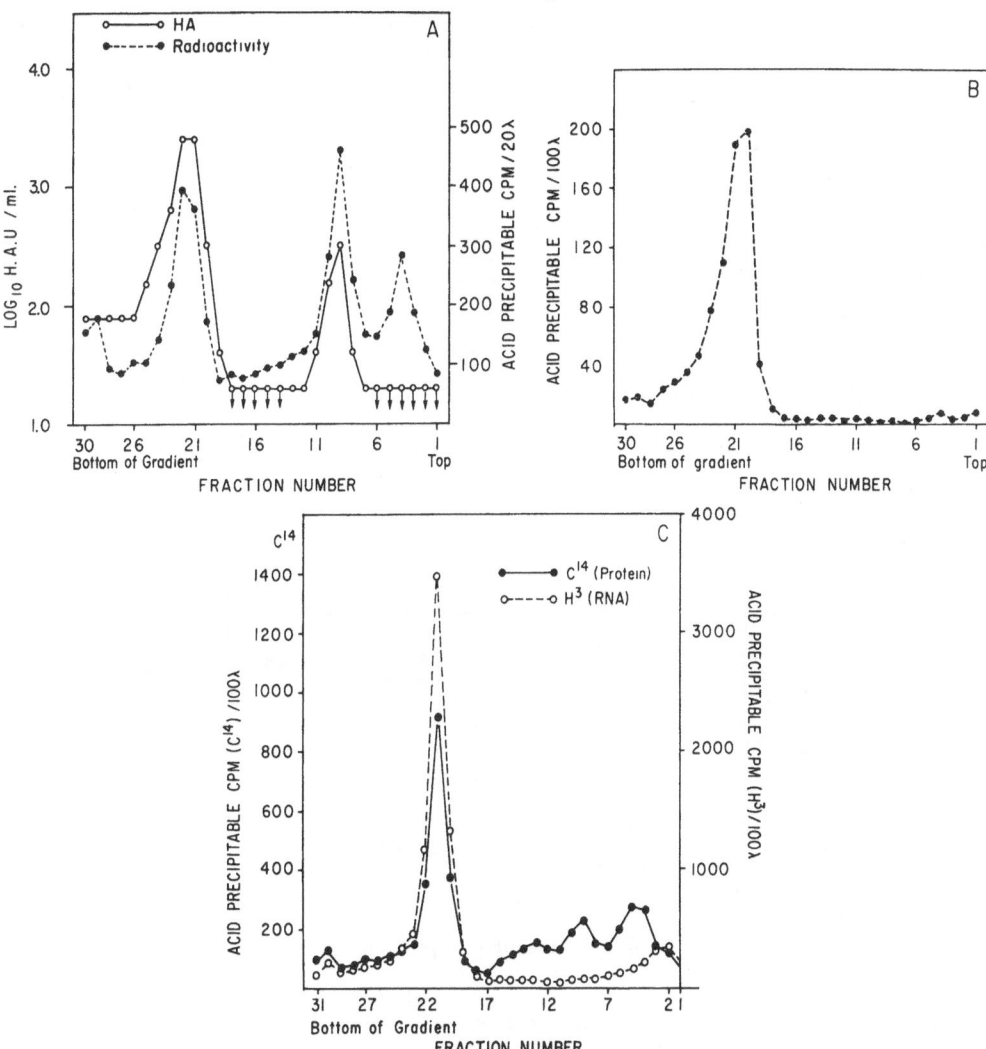

Fig. 11. Sucrose gradients of radioactively labeled dengue-2 virus.
(A) Sucrose gradient centrifugation of ^{14}C amino acid-labeled dengue-2 virus. The culture medium contained a mixture of ^{14}C amino acids (54 mCi/milliatom carbon) at concentrations of 0.1 μCi/ml from 1.5 to 24 hours and 1.0 μCi/ml from 24 to 48 hours after infection. The virus was concentrated by ultracentrifugation and purified by sucrose gradient centrifugation. (B) Recentrifugation in a sucrose gradient of fractions 22 and 23 of the gradient shown in (A), pooled and diluted 1:5 in BABS 9. Of this diluted virus, 2.5 ml was examined by a second sucrose gradient centrifugation. Fractions were assayed for acid-precipitable radioactivity only. (C) Sucrose gradient centrifugation of uridine-^{3}H and $^{-14}$C mixed amino acid-labeled dengue-2 virus. Uridine-^{3}H (20 Ci/mmole) was present at concentrations of 1 μCi/ml from 1.5 to 24 hours and 5 μCi/ml from 24 to 48 hours after infection. ^{14}C-labeled amino acids (1 mCi/mg) were present at concentrations of 0.1 μCi/ml from 1.5 to 24 hours and 1 μCi/ml from 24 to 48 hours after infection. Virus was concentrated first by (NH$_4$)$_2$SO$_4$ precipitation and then by ultracentrifugation. Fractions were assayed for both ^{3}H and ^{14}C acid-precipitable radioactivity. From STOLLAR (1969)
With permission of the author and Academic Press, Inc., New York

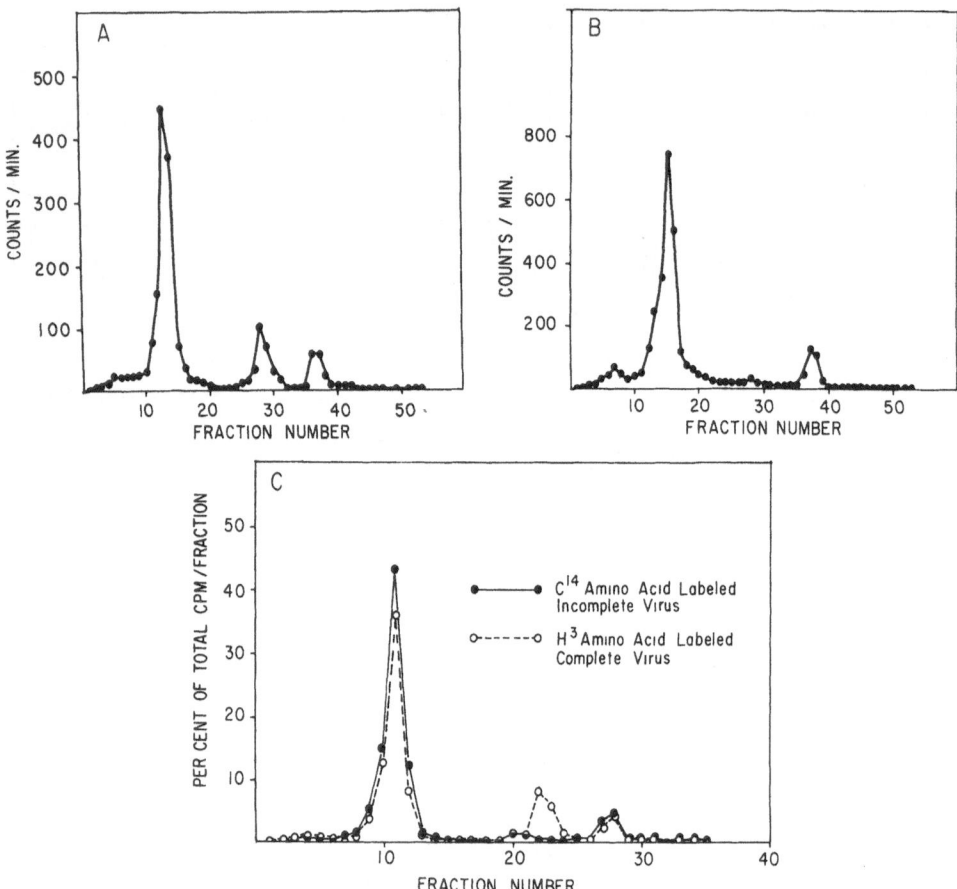

Fig. 12. Gel electrophoreses of proteins of complete (RHA) and incomplete (SHA)
dengue-2 virus.
(A) Acrylamide gel electrophoresis of ^{14}C amino acid-labeled complete virus. A portion
of the complete virus peak shown in Fig. 11A was treated with SDS-mercaptoethanol
and subjected to acrylamide gel electrophoresis. Fractions were collected every
15 seconds using the Savant gel extruder. (B) Acrylamide gel electrophoresis of ^{14}C
amino acid-labeled incomplete virus. A portion of the incomplete virus peak shown in
Fig. 11A was treated with SDS-mercaptoethanol and examined by acrylamide gel
electrophoresis. Fractions were collected every 15 seconds. (C) Acrylamide gel electrophoresis of ^{14}C amino acid-labeled incomplete virus and ^{3}H amino acid-labeled complete
virus. A ^{14}C-labeled protein hydrolyzate (54 mCi/milliatom carbon) was used to
prepare ^{14}C-labeled virus. ^{14}C amino acids were present at concentrations of 0.1 μCi/ml
from 1.5 to 24 hours and 0.6 μCi/ml from 24 to 48 hours after infection. Mixed ^{3}H-
labeled amino acids were used to prepare ^{3}H-labeled virus. ^{3}H amino acids were present
at concentrations of 1 μCi/ml from 1.5 to 24 hours and 8.5 μCi/ml from 24 to 48 hours
after infection. The ^{14}C-labeled virus was concentrated by $(NH_4)_2SO_4$ precipitation
followed by ultracentrifugation, while the ^{3}H-labeled virus was concentrated by
ultracentrifugation alone. Each virus preparation was purified by sucrose gradient
centrifugation. The appropriate peaks were taken from each gradient, treated with
SDS-mercaptoethanol, mixed and examined by acrylamide gel electrophoresis
From STOLLAR (1969). With permission of the author and Academic Press, Inc.,
New York

cells in the presence of ^{14}C-amino acids (Fig. 11a). Recentrifugation of the "complete" virus peak reveals its homogeneity and failure to shift to the position of "incomplete" virus (Fig. 11b). Moreover, double-labeling with ^{14}C-amino acids and ^{3}H-uridine shows coincidence of the RNA and protein labels only in the "complete" component of the gradient (Fig. 11c) (STOLLAR, 1969).

Polyacrylamide gel electrophoresis (PAGE) of appropriate sucrose gradient fractions, degraded with sodium dodecyl sulfate (SDS) and mercaptoethanol according to SUMMERS et al. (1965), has resulted in the patterns illustrated in Fig. 12. In order of their electrophoretic migration, the three polypeptide peaks associated with "complete" virions have been identified as VP-1, -2, -3 (reading from right to left in Fig. 12a). As shown in Fig. 12b, "incomplete" virus lacks demonstrable amounts of VP-2, and this is borne out by co-electrophoresis of ^{3}H-labeled "complete" and ^{14}C-labeled "incomplete" virus from the same gradient (Fig. 12c). The prominence of VP-2 in that portion of the viral population which contains $>90\%$ of the 45S viral RNA and of the infectivity strongly suggests that VP-2 is the "core" protein associated with the viral genome.

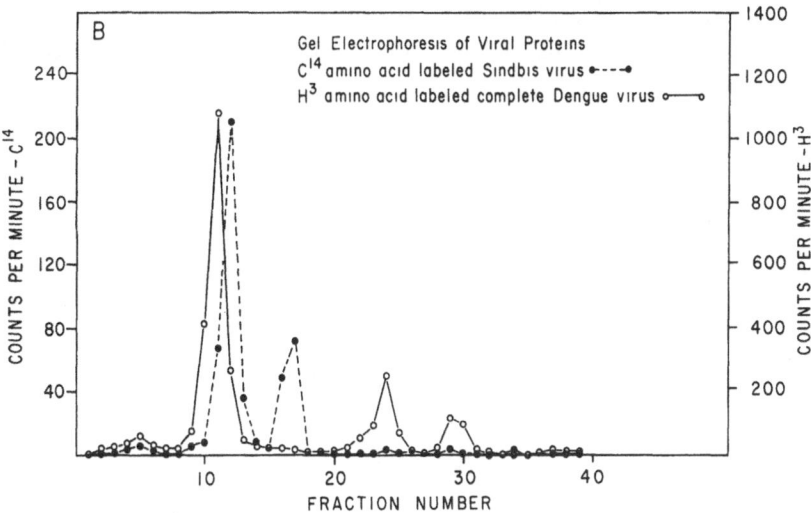

Fig. 13. Acrylamide gel co-electrophoresis of ^{14}C amino acid-labeled Sindbis virus and ^{3}H amino acid-labeled "complete" dengue virus. From STOLLAR (1969) With permission of the author and Academic Press, Inc., New York

The finding of at least 3 polypeptides of distinct sizes in infectious dengue-2 virions marks a contrast to Sindbis virus for which STRAUSS et al. (1968) originally reported only 2 polypeptides (MW 30,000 for the "core" protein, 53,000 for the envelope glycoprotein, STRAUSS et al., 1969). Co-electrophoresis of ^{14}C amino acid-labeled Sindbis and ^{3}H amino acid-labeled "complete" dengue-2 virus confirms this distinction (Fig. 13) and permits an estimate of the molecular weights of the three dengue-2 polypeptides as 7,700 for VP-1, 13,500 for VP-2, 59,000 for VP-3. M. J. SCHLESINGER et al. (1972) have resolved the Sindbis virion envelope into two glycoproteins (E1 and 2), of similar molecular weights but different peptide composition, by a discontinuous SDS PAGE system. They have also identified a precursor glycoprotein to E2 *i.e.*, PE2 (S. SCHLESINGER and M. J. SCHLESINGER. 1972). GAROFF *et al.* (1974) identified a third glycoprotein, E3 (MW 10.000.

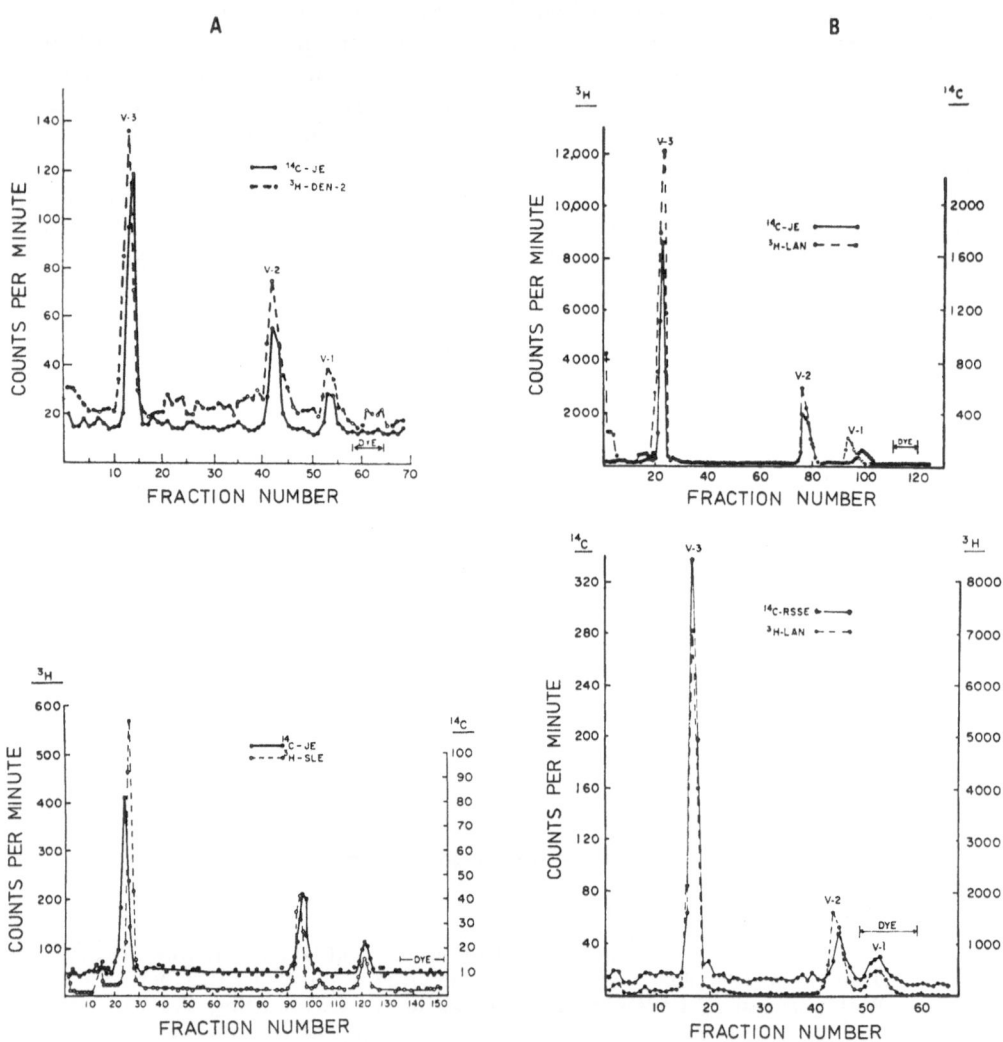

Fig. 14. Acrylamide gel electrophoresis of structural polypeptides of mosquito- and tick-borne group B togaviruses: Each panel presents co-electrophoresis of one ¹⁴C- and one ³H-amino acid-labeled virus

Mosquito-borne viruses   JE—Japanese encephalitis
                                  DEN 2—dengue-2
                                  SLE—St. Louis encephalitis
Tick-borne viruses   LAN—Langat
                                  RSSE—Russian spring-summer encephalitis
For further details see SHAPIRO *et al.* (1972d)
Modified from SHAPIRO *et al.* (1972d). With permission of the authors and the American Society for Microbiology

containing 45% carbohydrate), in Semliki forest virions. No evidence has been adduced to date which would suggest resolution of more than one glycoprotein in dengue or other group B togavirions (PFEFFERKORN and SHAPIRO, 1974). However, it has been suggested by SHAPIRO et al. (1972b) that a glycosylated polypeptide (NV2) found in dengue-2 virions released from cells maintained in Tris buffer may be a precursor of the non-glycosylated envelope polypeptide VP-1. More about these relationships in Section VIII. D. (Morphogenesis).

Results analogous to those cited above for dengue-2 virus have been reported for various other group B togaviruses (WESTAWAY and REEDMAN, 1969; TRENT and QURESHI, 1971; SHAPIRO et al., 1971; ROSATO et al., 1974; WESTAWAY, 1973, 1975) except for somewhat variable estimates of the MW of VP-3 (53,000—59,000) and VP-1 (7,700—9,000). Of special interest is the finding (SHAPIRO et al., 1972d) of very closely similar PAGE mobility for the polypeptides of five *mosquito*-borne group B togaviruses, including dengue-2 (Fig. 14a). Four *tick*-borne group B togaviruses likewise resembled each other closely with regard to their polypeptides, but the mobility of VP-1 was consistently lower for the latter than for the mosquito-borne viruses (Fig. 14b). This may be a valuable biochemical clue to the evolutionary distinctness of these subgroups.

Table 7. *Relative incorporation of radioactive amino acids into the proteins of dengue-2 virus*[a]

Label	Gradient fractions	VP-3, MW 59,000	VP-2, MW 13,500	VP-4, MW 7,700
Mixed amino acids-[14]C	RHA	100	20.5	12.2
	SHA	100	4.0	12.8
Methionine-[14]C	RHA	100	27.6	10.0
	SHA	100	6.2	12.2
Lysine-[14]C	RHA	100	29.5	2.3
	SHA	100	7.0	3.6
Histidine-[14]C	RHA	100	< 2.0	20.1
	SHA	100	< 2.0	27.2
Methionine-[35]S	RHA	100	28.7	11.7
	NP 40 light fractions	100	5.9	10.0

[a] In each experiment the number of counts in VP-3 was set as equal to 100, and from the counts in each of the other 2 peaks, the values were calculated for VP-1 and VP-2 relative to VP-3.
Modified from STOLLAR (1969).

Further insight into the nature, possible function and distribution within the virion of the three dengue-2 polypeptides has come from the labeling of KB cell-grown virus with single amino acids. The results of such experiments (STOLLAR, 1969) are summarized in Table 7. It is evident that (a) the distribution of [14]C- or ^{35}S-methionine label among the 3 polypeptides closely resembles that obtained with mixed radioactive amino acids; (b) lysine is incorporated much more prominently into VP-2 than -1, possibly consistent with the nature of VP-2 as a (basic?)

RNA-associated protein; (c) no incorporation of radioactive histidine into VP-2 is demonstrable, a feacture of special interest in view of the reported absence of histidine from the capsid proteins of RNA bacteriophages (OHTAKA and SPIEGELMAN, 1963) and tobacco mosaic virus (cf. FRAENKEL-CONRAT. 1968); (d) regardless of the nature of the amino acid label incorporated. the ratio (VP-3/VP-1) is similar for "complete" (RHA) and "incomplete" (SHA) virus; (e) the reduction of VP-2 in "incomplete" virus is similarly reflected in terms of mixed amino acid, methionine. or lysine label incorporated in this component. In addition, STOLLAR (1969) has shown that ^{14}C-glucosamine is incorporated only into VP-3, indicating that it is a glycoprotein.

Finally, degradation of gradient-purified "complete" dengue-2 virus, labeled in RNA with ^{3}H-uridine and in protein with ^{14}C-mixed amino acids. with the non-ionic detergent Nonidet-P40 leads to the separation of a "core", containing about 10% of the ^{14}C and all of the ^{3}H label. from a component near the top of the gradient containing 90% of the ^{14}C label (Fig. 15). Acrylamide gel electrophoresis shows that the "core" contains only VP-2 while the "light" component resembles in polypeptide composition the naturally occurring "incomplete" virus (bottom of Table 7) (STOLLAR. 1969).

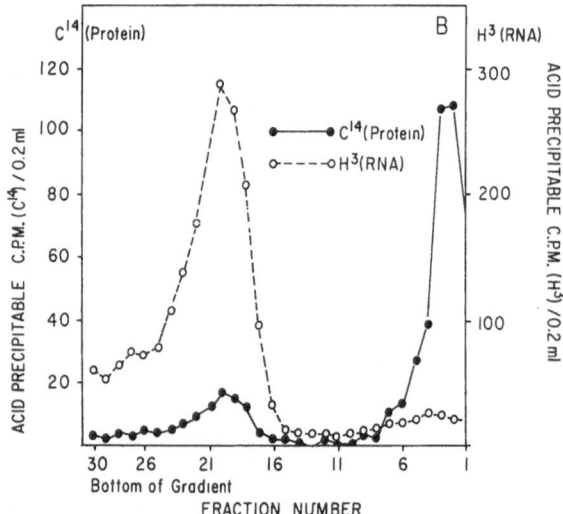

Fig. 15. NP-40 treatment of dengue-2 virus. Sucrose gradient centrifugation of NP-40-treated and ^{3}H-uridine ^{14}C amino acid-labeled "complete" virus.
A portion of complete virus (RHA) from the sucrose gradient shown in Fig. 11C was treated with NP-40. Centrifugation was at 25,000 rpm for 3.25 hours in the SW 25.1 rotor. Fractions were assayed for both ^{3}H and ^{14}C acid-precipitable radioactivity.
From STOLLAR (1969)
With permission of the author and Academic Press, Inc.. New York

These findings invite the following interpretations: (a) VP-3, a glycoprotein. is the major envelope protein; (b) VP-2 is associated with the RNA "core", and presumably represents the capsid protein; (c) VP-1 is associated with the envelope and could possibly represent a second envelope protein, comparable to the "M" polypeptide of myxoviruses (cf. SCHULZE, 1973). It should be noted, however, that VP-1 remains associated with "cores" of JEV and Kunjin if the virions are dissociated with deoxycholate instead of nonionic detergents (WESTAWAY and REEDMAN, 1969; WESTAWAY, 1973).

Together with a fourth antigenically virus-specific polypeptide (the soluble CF antigen, a non-structural protein, MW 39,000 daltons; see Section VI. E. 1.), these viral proteins would account for about 25% of the coding capacity of a viral genome of 4.2 million dalton.

4. Carbohydrates

The monosaccharides associated with the envelope glycoprotein VP-3 of dengue virus have not been analyzed. Japanese encephalitis virus has been reported to contain glucosamine, galactose, mannose, and fucose (SHAPIRO et al., 1973a), and it is likely that dengue viruses would be similar. Nothing has been reported about the presence of sialic acid in group B togaviruses. This would be of special interest in comparison with Sindbis virus which does contain it in varying amounts depending on the vertebrate cells in which it has been grown (STRAUSS et al., 1970), but not when it is isolated from mosquito cells which lack sialic acid in their membrane glycoproteins (STOLLAR et al., 1975). Inasmuch as the envelope of Sindbis and other group A togaviruses are derived from cellular plasma membrane while those of the group B viruses are thought to originate within the cytoplasm (see Section VII. A. 6. on Morphogenesis), the presence or absence of sialic acid in the latter viruses may provide interesting information concerning the biogenesis of cytoplasmic membranes.

D. Biological Activities of Viral Components

1. Infectious Viral RNA

ADA and ANDERSON (1959), NAKAMURA (1961), and SCHULZE (1962) demonstrated independently that phenol extracts of dengue-1 or -2 infected mouse brains contained ribonuclease-sensitive, infectious material. The intracerebral

Table 8. *Infectivity of dengue-2 viral RNA*[a]

Method of assay	PFU/ml[b]	EOP $\dfrac{\text{RNA}^c}{\text{Virus}}$
DEAE-dextran	1.4×10^4	4.2×10^{-5}
Hypertonic saline	6.8×10^3	2.1×10^{-5}
DEAE-dextran and hypertonic saline	3.3×10^5	1.0×10^{-3}
RNase-treated[d], DEAE-dextran and hypertonic saline	$< 10^2$	—

[a] Extracted from stock virus containing 3.3×10^8 PFU/ml.
[b] Corrected for change in volume from that of initial virus suspension.
[c] Efficiency of plating of RNA relative to that of initial virus suspension (3.3×10^8 PFU/ml).
[d] Two micrograms per milliliter, 15 minutes at 20°.

Modified from STOLLAR et al. (1967).

titer of this "RNA" ranged from 10^{-4} to 10^{-6} of the LD_{50} contained in the untreat-ed, RNase-resistant starting material. Subsequently, STOLLAR et al. (1967) extracted RNA from virus grown in KB cell cultures and assayed its plaque-forming ability. As shown in Table 8, maximum efficiency of plating (EOP) relative to the original viral titer was obtained when washing of the BHK-21 assay cells with hypertonic salt solution was combined with addition of DEAE-dextran to the RNA.

The intrinsic infectiousness of dengue virion RNA indicates, by definition (BALTIMORE, 1971), that it is of "plus" (messenger) polarity. One would therefore not expect to find virion-associated RNA polymerase, but direct tests have not yet been reported.

2. Hemagglutinating "Subunits"

A "soluble" HA (SHA) has been separated from rapidly sedimenting viral particles (RHA) by sucrose gradient centrifugation of dengue-2 infected mouse brain extract (SMITH et al., 1970). The SHA particle appears, in negatively stained preparations, as a "doughnut" structure with a diameter of 13.8 to 14 nm and a central "hole" 5 to 7 nm in diameter. No comparable configuration can be discerned on the surface of intact virions, and therefore the positioning and shape of the HA subunit in the viral particles (RHA) remains in doubt. By analogy with other enveloped viruses (including group A togaviruses), it is likely that the attachment to RBC is mediated by a surface component carrying the envelope-associated glycoprotein VP-3, and that this, in turn, forms part of the spikes or knobs projecting from the viral envelope in electron micrographs.

On the other hand, disruption of virions by ether or deoxycholate leads to loss of HA as well as of infectivity, suggesting that total loss of viral lipids may not be compatible with retention of HA activity. This impression is borne out by the fact (STEVENS and SCHLESINGER, unpublished) that treatment of gradient-purified dengue-2 virus with a mixture of Tween 80 and ethyl ether leads to a net increase in HA activity and yields an immunologically specific HA split product which sediments in sucrose gradients in the same velocity range as "incomplete" virus. However, in CsCl equilibrium density gradients, it bands at a density of about 1.27 g/ml, i.e., heavier than "complete" virions. This density would be expected of a protein fragment of the envelope still associated with some (but significantly reduced) lipids. Such a structural arrangement would be required if each HA subunit had only one attachment site and the lipid were needed to hold together dimers or polymers of such subunits and thus form an effective bridge between two erythrocytes. The SHA subviral particle of SMITH et al. (1970), described above, has a density in CsCl of 1.23 g/ml, indicating considerable lipid contents along with the (presumed) HA glycoprotein.

E. Antigenic Structure

Although a massive volume of literature has been published on the immunologic relationships of dengue types to each other and to other group B togaviruses, only a few recent studies are helpful in attempting to relate individual antigens to known structural and chemical features of the virion itself. Although the issue is confused, a review is important because of the strong indication that clear delineation of antigenic relationships extending to *all* group B togaviruses *(group-specific)* or only to the dengue viruses *(subgroup-specific)* from those that are strictly *type-specific* (for dengue-1, *or -2, or -3, or -4*) holds the key to an understanding of pathogenic mechanisms in secondary infections (see Section X. C.).

1. Group-Specific Antigens

The nature of the evidence leading to the assignment of dengue viruses to the group B togaviruses has been summarized in Section IV. It is based mainly on the extensive cross reactions, in HI and CF tests, among all members of this large group (SWEET and SABIN, 1954; CASALS and BROWN, 1954; SABIN and YOUNG, 1949). By analogy to the myxoviruses (where *"type"* corresponds, in accepted usage, to *"group"* as used for togaviruses), one might expect the common antigen to be associated with the nucleocapsid of the virion, more unique antigens forming part of the viral envelope (cf. HOYLE, 1968). The validity of this analogy is suggested by studies on group A togaviruses (Sindbis, Eastern and Western equine encephalomyelitis virus) in which "envelope" and "core" components were separated from virions by treatment with Nonidet-P40 (see Section VI. C. 3.) and examined by reciprocal radioimmune precipitation (DALRYMPLE *et al.*, 1973). Whole viruses or purified "envelope" material showed limited cross reactions between Sindbis and WEE viruses but none between these two and EEE virus. In contrast, the "core" preparations cross-reacted extensively.

In the case of the group B togaviruses, this approach has not yet been as fully applied, and relatively little work has been done with fractionated and rigorously characterized immunogens or antigens derived from purified virions. The extensive cross-reactions observed in HI tests suggest that a common antigen is associated with the envelope.

This has indeed been demonstrated by WESTAWAY *et al.* (1975) who showed extensive reciprocal cross-inhibition of HA by three group B viruses, including dengue-2, by their respective immune sera. The cross-reactivity in HI tests resided entirely in the IgG fraction of immune sera, while the IgM fraction was type-specific (see below).

QURESHI and TRENT (1973a, b) used the major envelope protein (their "Antigen I") isolated from extracts of cells infected with SLE, JBE, WN, or dengue-2 viruses in CF tests with homologous or heterologous *antiviral* hyperimmune mouse ascitic fluids. They observed extensive cross-reactivity among the first three viruses, less or none between them and dengue-2 (although it should be noted that both antigen and antibody titers in homologous tests with the latter system were significantly lower than in any of the other systems, hence presumably less sensitive in detecting possible cross-reactions).

In working with crude whole virus preparations as antigens, obscuring of type- or subgroup-specific complement-fixation reactions by group B cross reaction can be minimized by use of hyperimmune mouse ascitic fluids (SARTORELLI *et al.*, 1965) rather than sera from hyperimmunized animals (TIKASINGH *et al.*, 1966; BRANDT *et al.*, 1967), although the same fluids are broadly reactive in the HI test. CLARKE (1960) showed earlier that absorption of broadly reactive dengue-1 and -2 immune sera with West Nile virus effectively removed group-reactive HI antibody but left dengue subgroup or type-specific antibodies only moderately diminished. Close topical relationship between type-, subgroup-, and group-specific antigens is further suggested by the fact that sera of human beings or of animals that have been exposed sequentially to more than one group B togavirus cross-react with different members of the group not only in CF and HI but also in neutralization tests (see Sections X and XI). To sum up, a strong case can be made for group- as well as type-(and subgroup-)specific determinants on the envelope gylcoprotein. The latter (VP-3) is the principal antigen involved in neutralization (cf. PFEFFERKORN and SHAPIRO, 1974) and hemagglutination inhibition.

Several investigators have shown that the cross-reactive immunoglobulin in sera after multiple infections is IgG while the IgM fraction is specifically reactive with the recent challenge virus (WESTAWAY, 1968; WESTAWAY *et al.*, 1974, 1975; EDELMAN and PARIYANONDA, 1973; SCOTT *et al.*, 1972).

The situation is further complicated by the fact that "incomplete" (SHA) and "complete" (RHA) dengue-2 virus (see Sections VI. B. 3. and VI. D. 2.) differ not only in polypeptide profile but, according to CARDIFF *et al.* (1971), also in antigenic specificity. A polypeptide associated with SHA appears to be identical to the (non-virion) glycoprotein (NV-2) which has been suggested as a precursor to envelope protein VP-1 (SHAPIRO *et al.*, 1972 b). This will be discussed more fully in Section VII.

On the other hand, WESTAWAY *et al.* (1975) have been unable to distinguish RHA from SHA by HI tests with antisera prepared against purified viral envelope antigens.

Nevertheless, it should be recognized that the morphogenetic scheme proposed for group B togaviruses by SHAPIRO *et al.* (1972 b) would mean that infected or actively immunized permissive hosts are exposed to the immunogenic stimulus not only of mature virion antigens but also of putative membrane precursor antigen(s). It will be interesting to learn if the latter are more crossreactive among all group B togaviruses than the virion ("RHA")-associated antigens.

2. Subgroup (Dengue)-Specific Antigens

As was pointed out in Section IV (Classification), the immunological basis for separating the dengue viruses from other (non-dengue) group B togaviruses has been elusive. Their designation as a distinct subgroup has rested primarily on clinical and other biological (host and vector spectrum) criteria, usually combined with the presence of group- and type-specific antigens. The existence of (additional?) subgroup-specific determinants (cf. earlier results of SMITHBURN, 1954 and others) was reexamined by DE MADRID and PORTERFIELD (1974). They tested each of 42 group B togaviruses for plaque neutralization against each of the corresponding 42 rabbit immune sera. There were 6 viruses which showed only homospecific neutralization. The remainder fell into seven subgroups within each of which there was extensive cross-neutralization. *The 4 dengue types constituted one of the subgroups, with no overlap into any of the others.* The validity of this subgroup designation is borne out, by inference, by the apparent role of subgroup-specific immunological phenomena involved in the dengue hemorrhagic fever and shock syndrome (see Section X) and by the finding that the "memory" of IgM (as measured by HI) asserts itself only when challenge of previously immunized animals involves a virus of the same subgroup as the primary one (WESTAWAY et al., 1974).

3. Type- and Strain-Specific Antigens

The recognition of at least four antigenically distinct types of dengue viruses is most readily accomplished by neutralization tests. Although the characterization of prototype strains belonging to these four types was initially based mainly on evaluation of "neutralization indices" (see critique in Section V.), more refined tests have borne out this differentiation. Key steps in the confirmation of these results are summarized in Tables 9—12, starting with the initial experiments in human volunteers by SABIN (1950). Included in Table 12 are data on the two strains (TH-36 and TH-SMAN) isolated by HAMMON et al. (1960a, b; 1961) from cases of dengue hemorrhagic fever in Thailand which these authors originally suggested as possible candidate prototype strains of types 5 and 6. The basis for their proposal was the finding that primary human convalescent sera (but not sera from immunized animals) usually permitted a distinction to be made between these two strains and closely related type 2 and 1 prototype strains (HAMMON and SATHER, 1964a, b). The limitations of this interpretation were suggested by the failure of plaque neutralization tests to distinguish TH-36 from type 2 or TH-SMAN from type 1 (Table 12). Moreover, it has been found repeatedly that individual strains of dengue-2 or -4 virus, isolated from patients or mosquitoes during localized outbreaks, show significant variations in the extent of plaque neutralization by a single prototype reference immune serum (e.g., RUSSELL et al., 1968, 1969). Similar studies on dengue-2 and -3 strains isolated during the Caribbean epidemics from 1963 to 1968 and on dengue-2 isolated in Nigeria in 1966 indicate that the dengue-2 strains are all closely related to those originating in Asia, while some of the type 3 strains from the Caribbean as well as one from Tahiti (ROSEN, 1967) show relatively poor cross neutralization with Southeast Asian prototype strains and thus seem to constitute bona fide subtypes (RUSSELL and McCOWN, 1972). Such variations could explain the apparent differences in the extent of plaque neutralization between type 1 and 2 and the TH-SMAN and TH-36 strains reported by IBRAHIM et al. (1968c).

Table 9. *Differentiation of dengue-1 and -2 strains by dermal neutralization tests in human volunteers*[a]

Strain of virus	Type designation	Normal serum	Skin lesion resulting from mixture with				
			Human convalescent serum				
			Hawaii	NG "A"	NG "B"	NG "C"	NG "D"
Hawaii	1	+	0	0	+	+	+
New Guinea "A"	1	+	0	0	+	+	+
New Guinea "B"	2	+	+	+	0	0	0
New Guinea "C"	2	+	+	+	0	0	0
New Guinea "D"	2	+	+ ?	+	0	0	0

[a] From SABIN (1950). With permission of the author and the American Society for Microbiology

Table 10. *Differentiation of mouse-adapted dengue-1 and -2 viruses by neutralization tests with homotypic and heterotypic immune sera*

Exp. No.	Serum[a]			Virus[b]			
	Donor	Immunizing dengue strain[c]	Time interval between inoculation and bleeding (Mos.)	Dengue New Guinea B		Dengue Hawaii	
				LD_{50} (log)	Neutr. index	LD_{50} (log)	Neutr. index
I	Normal guinea pig	—	—	7.1 } 7.1	—	7.0 } 7.1	—
	Normal rabbit (10%)	—	—	7.0		7.1	
	Rhesus #27	New Guinea B	0[d]	6.8	2	7.0	0
			1	4.2	800	>6.4	<4
			3	3.2	8,000	>6.5	<3
			6	2.6	30,000	>6.5	<3
	Rhesus #28	Hawaii	0[d]	7.4	0	6.5	3
			1	n.t.	n.t.	5.2	64
			3	>6.5	<4	3.7	2,000
			6	5.8	20	3.8	1,600
II	Normal guinea pig	—	—	7.4	—	6.6	—
	Rhesus #29	New Guinea D	0[d]	7.5	0	6.4	2
			1	6.1	20	5.8	6
			6	4.3	1,300	6.0	4
III	Normal guinea pig	—	—	6.7	—	6.4	—
	Rhesus #569[e]	New Guinea B	1	3.8	800	6.0	3
	Rhesus #934[e]	New Guinea C	1.3	4.3	250	5.4	10
	Rhesus #936[e]	New Guinea C	1.3	4.7	100	5.5	8
	Rhesus #570[e]	New Guinea D	1.5	4.2	320	5.7	5
	Rhesus #28	Hawaii	6	6.6	0	3.0	2,500
IV	Normal guinea pig	—	—	6.8	—	6.5	—
	Patient W. H. convalescent	New Guinea B	2	<3.6	>1,600	5.5	10

[a] All sera were heated at 56° C for 30 minutes and diluted 1:4 before addition of equal parts of unheated normal guinea pig serum. Hence, the neutralization indices are those of 1:8 diluted sera.

[b] Viruses were used in the form of infected baby mouse brain suspensions.

[c] All immunizations were done by intracerebral inoculation of 1.0 ml of human acute phase sera.

[d] Serum obtained immediately prior to inoculation.

[e] These sera were kindly supplied by Dr. A. B. Sabin, Cincinnati.

n.t. Not tested.

From SCHLESINGER and FRANKEL (1952a). With permission of the American Journal of Tropical Medicine and Hygiene

Table 11. *Differentiation of 4 dengue types by neutralization tests in mice*[a]

Virus type	Neutralization index with antiserum against type			
	1	2	3	4
1	5400	170	160	140
2	10	1000	72	27
3	4	2	1000	3
4	4	2	1	>4350

[a] Based on HAMMON *et al.* (1960a). With permission of the author and Science (Copyright 1960 by the American Association for the Advancement of Science).

Table 12. *Differentiation of dengue types by plaque neutralization*[a]

Virus strains	Type designation	50% plaque reduction titer of monkey immune serum against					
		1	2	3	4	TH-36	TH-Sman
Hawaii	1	*300*	<10	90	10	<10	*100*
New Guinea „C"	2	<10	*1400*	30	13	*1700*	<10
H-87	3	<10	<10	*350*	<10	<10	<10
H-241	4	<10	<10	14	*150*	<10	<10
TH-36	2	<10	*2500*	NT[b]	NT	*2500*	NT
TH-Sman	1	*70*	<10	NT	NT	<10	*115*

[a] Data from RUSSELL and NISALAK (1967). With permission of the authors and the Williams & Wilkins Co., Baltimore
[b] Not tested.

Conflicting findings have also been reported for immunodiffusion experiments. CHAN (1965) reported highly specific Ouchterlony reactions of types 1, 2, 3, and 4 with their respective homologous immune sera only. Although both reactants were crude, only single bands of precipitation were seen. HAWKES and MARSHALL (1967) suggested that "dengue antigens displayed a high degree of specificity in the gel-diffusion reaction . . .". Immunoelectrophoresis was used by CUADRADO and CASALS (1967) who came to the conclusion that HT-36 was indistinguishable from dengue-2, and TH-SMAN from dengue-1. Their result was questioned by IBRAHIM and HAMMON (1968a, b) on technical grounds and on the basis of their own evidence in immunoelectrophoresis and gel double diffusion experiments. The latter revealed that two or three bands of precipitation, characteristic of heterotypic cross reactions, could be reduced to 1 or 2 bands by appropriate cross-absorption of the immune sera. However, similar tests with multiple strains assigned to each of the four prototypes might have shown similar results. It is concluded that, as of this writing, only four major antigenic types of dengue virus have been clearly documented.

Despite to occurrence of group- or subgroup cross reactions in complement fixation (CF) (SABIN and YOUNG, 1949; SCHLESINGER and FRANKEL, 1952;

HAMMON and SATHER, 1964b) and in hemagglutination-inhibition (HI) tests
(SWEET and SABIN, 1954; CASALS and BROWN. 1954). titers of monospecific
homologous antisera are always higher than those obtained in heterologous reactions. Specificity in HI tests can be amplified by cross absorption (CLARKE. 1960)
or by fractionation of broadly reactive sera which reveals that IgG carries group-
and subgroup-specific determinants while IgM is type-specific (WESTAWAY. 1968:
SCOTT et al., 1972; EDELMAN and PARIYANONDA. 1973; WESTAWAY et al.. 1974,
1975).

The antigenic complexity of these viruses is obvious and, as discussed in
Section X, of immense medical importance because the coexistence of type-
specific and subgroup-specific determinants on the virions of different serotypes
provides the most plausible explanation of the disastrous complications of secondary
dengue, i.e., hemorrhagic fever and the shock syndrome. Much intensive work
is therefore needed to identify the structural subunit(s) carrying the different
antigens and the evolutionary pressures that are responsible for their differentiation.

4. Non-Structural Dengue Antigens

A soluble type-specific CF (SCF) antigen present in virus-infected tissues or cell
cultures was first described by BRANDT et al. (1969). Despite the non-structural
nature of this antigen, it is mentioned in the context of this discussion of virion
antigens because the variable presence of this material in crude antigen preparations, and of antibodies directed against it in antiviral immune sera, may introduce
reactions spuriously thought to relate to the virions themselves. This material
was partially purified by $(NH_4)_2SO_4$ precipitation of protamine sulfate-treated.
dengue-infected mouse brain. It has no HA activity and, in contrast to the RHA
and SHA fractions, resists denaturation by sodium lauryl sulfate plus 2-mercapto-
ethanol (BRANDT et al., 1970). It has a buoyant density in CsCl of 1.32 g/ml.
Elution from Sephadex G-100 and polyacrylamide gel electrophoresis has suggested
a single polypeptide molecule of MW = 39,000 daltons, with different mobilities
for each type of dengue virus, indicating that they represent type-specific charge
isomers of a single molecule (CARDIFF et al., 1970). Detailed analysis of the physical
and antigenic properties of the SCF antigen from infected mouse brains has led to
the conclusion that it is a non-structural product, i.e., not incorporated into
mature virions (BRANDT et al., 1970). Immunoprecipitation analysis employing
hyperimmune ascitic fluids from mice immunized with crude infected mouse
brain suspensions has revealed an antigenic determinant common to all four
dengue serotypes which can be removed by cross absorption. In addition, there
is a type-specific component, and precipitation patterns indicate that both antigenic determinants are carried on the same molecule (RUSSELL et al., 1970).

McCLOUD et al. (1971) critically reexamined the interrelationships between
the Hawaii prototype 1 strain and the TH-SMAN strain on one hand and between
New Guinea "C" and TH-36 representing type 2 variants on the other, in terms
of the physical and immunological properties of their respective SCF antigens.
They concluded that the two type 2 strains could not be distinguished from each
other in terms of immunodiffusion, cross CF titrations, or disc gel electrophoresis
of the purified SCF antigens. On the other hand, minor differences were observed

between Hawaii and TH-SMAN antigens in terms of cross CF and electrophoretic mobility. These authors concluded that these subtle differences "may be sufficient to account for the original separation of the two dengue-1 strains".

Another non-structural antigen ("Antigen III") of MW 85,000 daltons has been solubilized from extracts of pig kidney (PS) cells infected with SLE, JE, WN, or dengue-2 viruses (QURESHI and TRENT, 1973a, b). This antigen is reported to react strictly specifically in CF and immunodiffusion tests with the homologous antiviral ascitic fluid. It is not clear, at the time of this writing, how this antigen relates to cell-associated polypeptides which have thus far been characterized by polyacrylamide gel electrophoresis, specifically NV-5 (see Table 15, Section VII. A. 5.).

F. Reactions to Physical and Chemical Agents

Dengue viruses appear to be relatively labile. However, the virus in the form of infective human serum can be preserved in the frozen or lyophilized state for long periods of time. The first report of this sort was published by HOFFMAN et al. (1932) who transported lyophilized patient's serum from Java to Amsterdam where its

Table 13. *Chemical inactivation of mouse or tissue culture passaged dengue viruses*

Agent	Original virus material[a]	Pre-treatment for purification of virus	Treatment for inactivation of infectivity	Authors
Ox bile	MB	—[b]	7%, 37°C, 2 hours, then 10°C, 24 hours	KIMURA and HOTTA (1944)
Deoxycholate	MB	Centrifugation (10,000 rpm)	0.1%, 37°C, 1 hour	THEILER (1957)
Acetone	MB	—	40%, 10 minutes	HASHIMOTO (1954)
Ethyl ether	MKTC	—	20%, 4°C, 24 hours	HOTTA and EVANS (1956c)
Lipase	HKTC	Cellulose column chromatography	125 unit/ml, pH 6.0, 30°C, 2 hours	TAKEHARA and HOTTA (1961)
Trypsin	MB	Protamine precipitation	0.5 mg/ml, pH 8.4, 37°C, 1 hour	HASHIMOTO (1955)
	MB	—	0.1%, pH 9.0, 37°C, 2 hours	GORMAN and GOSS (1972)
	HKTC	Cellulose column chromatography	0.125%, pH 7.2, 37°C, 2 hours	TAKEHARA and HOTTA (1961)
Chymotrypsin	MB	—	0.1%, pH 9.0, 37°C, 2 hours	GORMAN and GOSS (1972)
Pronase	MB	—	0.1%, pH 9.0, 37°C, 2 hours	GORMAN and GOSS (1972)

[a] MB   Mouse brain homogenate.
MKTC   Monkey kidney tissue culture fluid.
HKTC   Hamster kidney tissue culture fluid.
[b] Low speed centrifugation only.

infectivity was clearly demonstrated 285 days after lyophilization. Similar results were later obtained by several groups of investigators; *e.g.*, frozen or lyophilized human dengue virus in serum maintained infectivity for man during periods of up to 5 years (OGATA and YOSHII, 1943; OGATA and HASHIMOTO. 1944a; TODA *et al.*. 1944. 1946; SABIN, 1950. 1952a).

According to MANOUSSAKIS (1928), infective human dengue serum lost its infectivity upon heating at 50° C for 30 minutes. OGATA and YOSHII (1943) reported that the human dengue virus resisted exposure to ultrasonic waves (560 kilocycles per second) for 2 to 3 minutes. but was inactivated by the same action lasting for 15 to 30 minutes. SABIN (1952a) reported inactivation of infectivity as well as immunogenicity by ultraviolet irradiation or by treatment with 0.05 per cent formalin.

BLANC and CAMINOPETROS (1930) presented early data regarding resistance or sensitivity of human dengue virus to various chemical agents. Among their results. the inactivation by ox bile later proved to have an essential meaning.

These earlier investigations were conducted on human virus contained in serum from patients, and residual viral infectivity was tested by inoculating human volunteers. Therefore, the results are uncertain due to the protective effects of plasma proteins and the lack of quantitation.

More meaningful quantitative data have accumulated since introduction of the mouse and of *in vitro* cell cultures for propagation of dengue viruses. In

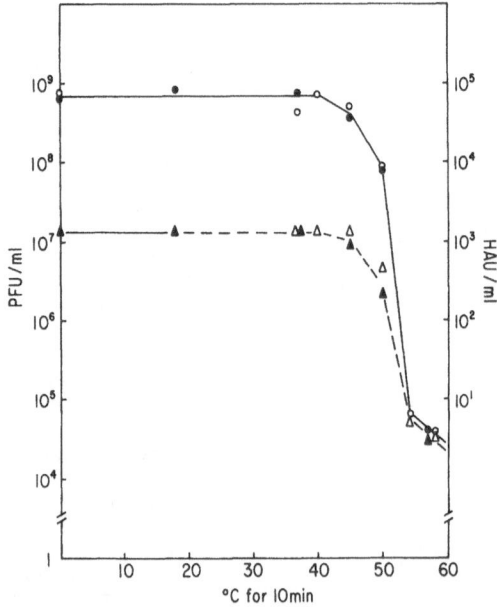

Fig. 16. Thermal inactivation of dengue-2 virus.
One ml aliquots of stock virus prepared from KB cell cultures infected with the New Guinea B strain of dengue-2 virus were incubated for 10 minutes at the indicated temperatures. Circles—infectivity assays; triangles—HA titrations. Open and closed symbols represent two separate experiments. T. M. STEVENS and V. STOLLAR. unpublished data

general, it has been the experience (largely unpublished) of investigators in this field that omission of some "protective" protein (*e.g.*, 0.2 per cent crystalline bovine albumin) from the suspending medium of purified virus leads to rapid loss of infectivity regardless of pH or temperature during storage. It is important to view the data summarized in Table 13 with this generally accepted fact in mind. All agents listed inactivate, presumably at similar rates, infectivity and HA activity. The parallelism of these responses of dengue-2 virus to *heat* inactivation is illustrated in Fig. 16.

Partially reversible complexing of dengue viruses with sulfated agar poly-saccharides leads to inhibition of HA as well as plaque-forming capacity (SCHULZE and SCHLESINGER, 1963b). SCHULZE (1964) studied quantitative aspects of this reaction in greater detail. Reversal could be achieved by dilution of the complex, and inhibition by the polyanion could be prevented by addition of polycations, especially soluble DEAE-dextran. Despite this evidence for direct interaction of the agar inhibitor with virus, use of cells other than KB (*e.g.*, Vero or LLC-MK2) can overcome the inhibitory effect (STIM, 1970b).

VII. Viral Replication in Cell Cultures

A. Vertebrate Cells

1. The Viral Growth Cycle

Adsorption of plaque-forming dengue-2 virus on KB cell monolayers follows essentially similar kinetics at 37° and at 28° C. At either temperature, the maximum number of PFU adsorbed is reached between 90 and 120 minutes after infection. However, it is reduced about 2-fold at the lower temperature (SCHULZE and SCHLESINGER, 1963a). According to STIM (1970a), adsorption is promoted by magnesium, reduced by calcium ions. The nature of cellular receptors has not been identified. The viral attachment site is likely to reside in the envelope glycoprotein (VP-3).

Nothing is known about the mechanism of penetration. The duration of the eclipse period is difficult to estimate because acquisition of infectiousness of newly produced virus appears to coincide with its release. Thus, the infectious titer of extracellular virus is always higher than that of cell-associated virus (see Section VII. A. 6., on Morphogenesis). After infection at multiplicities >5 PFU per cell, newly synthesized virus is first detected in the medium at 12—13 hours after infection (Fig. 17). The subsequent rises in PFU and HAU occur in parallel (SCHULZE, 1962, 1964; STEVENS *et al.*, 1962), remaining in any given experiment at a constant ratio ranging from 4.3 to 6.0 $\log_{10}$. The possible significance of this ratio in terms of physical particles as well as variables affecting its magnitude are discussed below (Section VII. C.). The increase in titer is exponential until about 24 hours after infection, then tapers off. From 30—36 hours onward, there is a gradual net decrease in virus released, but KB cell cultures under liquid medium can continue to liberate virus for years after initial infection (see below, persistently infected cells).

At the height of virus production, the yield at 37° C rarely exceeds an average of 200—500 PFU/cell. In contrast to the observation of HALLAUER and KRONAUER (1960) for yellow fever virus, no significant amounts of additional dengue-2 virus

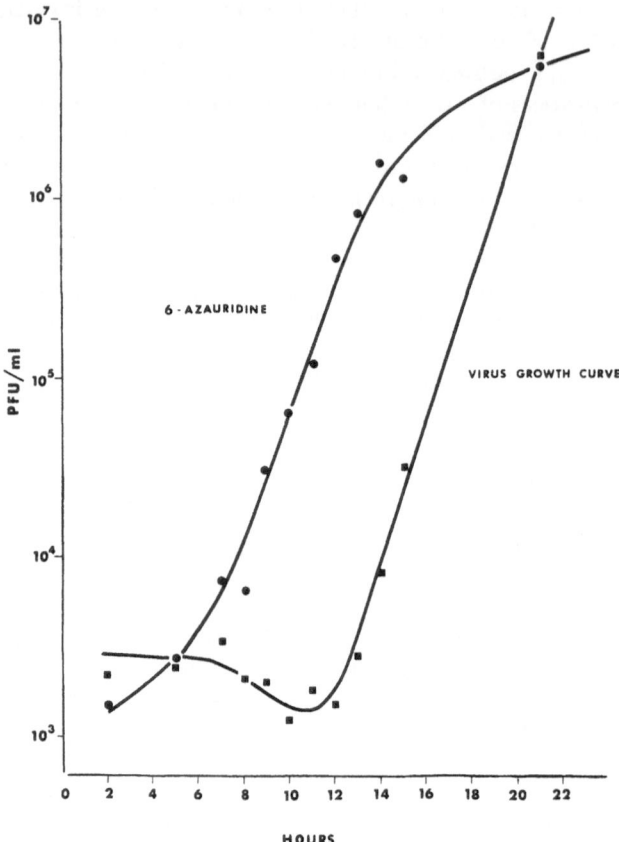

Fig. 17. Dengue-2 virus: One-step growth curve in KB cell monolayers and inhibition
of virus yield as a function of the time of addition of 6-azauridine.
At various times after infection, 6-azauridine was added (final concentration 5 µg/ml).
Virus was harvested from the medium of each treated culture at 24 hours after infection
and titrated for PFU. Modified from STOLLAR et al. (1966)

can be liberated from monolayer cultures by rinsing with alkaline borate buffer
(STEVENS and SCHLESINGER, 1965). It is, however, possible to achieve a significant
increase in the amount of virus released per cell by increasing the ionic strength
of the medium (see Section VII. D.).

The relatively low yields of dengue virus may be associated with sparse cell-
associated virions or viral precursors (cores) observable in electron micrographs
of infected KB or BHK-21 cells. Sometimes one finds only occasional virions in
cytoplasmic vacuoles and a few bodies of the electron density, shape, and size
expected of viral cores in the cytoplasm in close proximity to cytoplasmic membranes. Much greater accumulation of replicating dengue-2 virus is seen in simian
cell lines (VERO and LLC-MK 2) in the form of large crystalloid aggregates of
intracytoplasmic virions. However, the yield of *infectious* virus released from these
cells is usually lower than that from KB cells (MATSUMURA et al., 1971). Further
details will be discussed in Section VII. A. 6. (Morphogenesis).

2. Effects on Cells

a) Morphological Changes Associated With Virus Replication

Although several kinds of cultured vertebrate cells undergo cytopathic effects (CPE) upon infection with dengue viruses (see HOTTA, 1969; also Section V. B. 1.), histological and electron microscopic examinations have cast limited light on the specific nature of cytological damage. The CPE induced by dengue-2 virus in

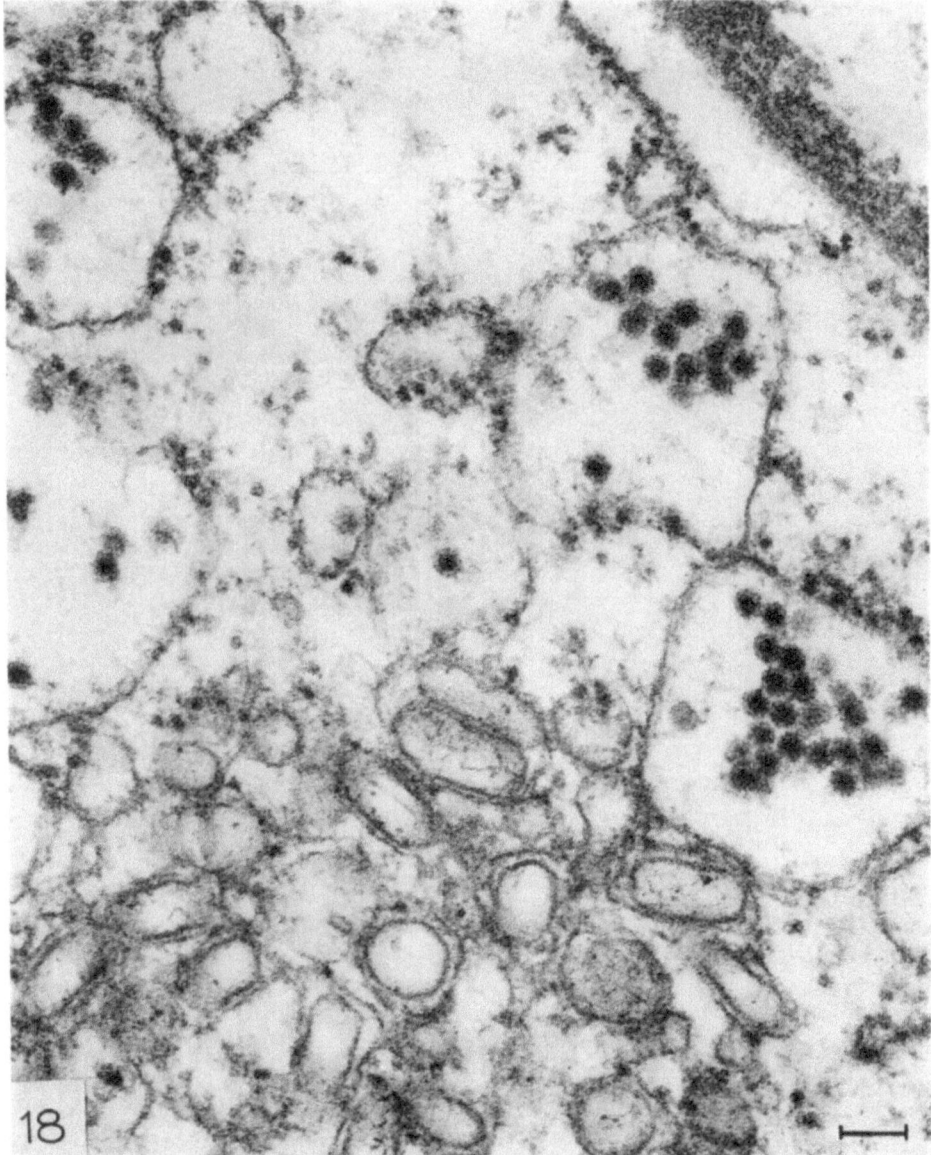

Fig. 18. Extensive vacuolization of cytoplasm in perinuclear region (nuclear membrane upper right) of dengue-2 virus-infected Vero cell, 24 hours after infection. Bar = 100 nm

human (KB), hamster (BHK-21), and simian cells consists in the main of more
or less pronounced cytoplasmic vacuolization. especially in the perinuclear zone.

Vero and LLC-MK 2 have been subjected to particularly detailed ultrastructural
analysis because massive cytoplasmic aggregates of virions can be demonstrated
in them (Matsumura et al.. 1971; Cardiff et al., 1973 b). The outstanding observable consequence of infection is progressive vacuolization of the cytoplasm
(Fig. 18). It is not clear whether this effect is due only to distension of pre-existing

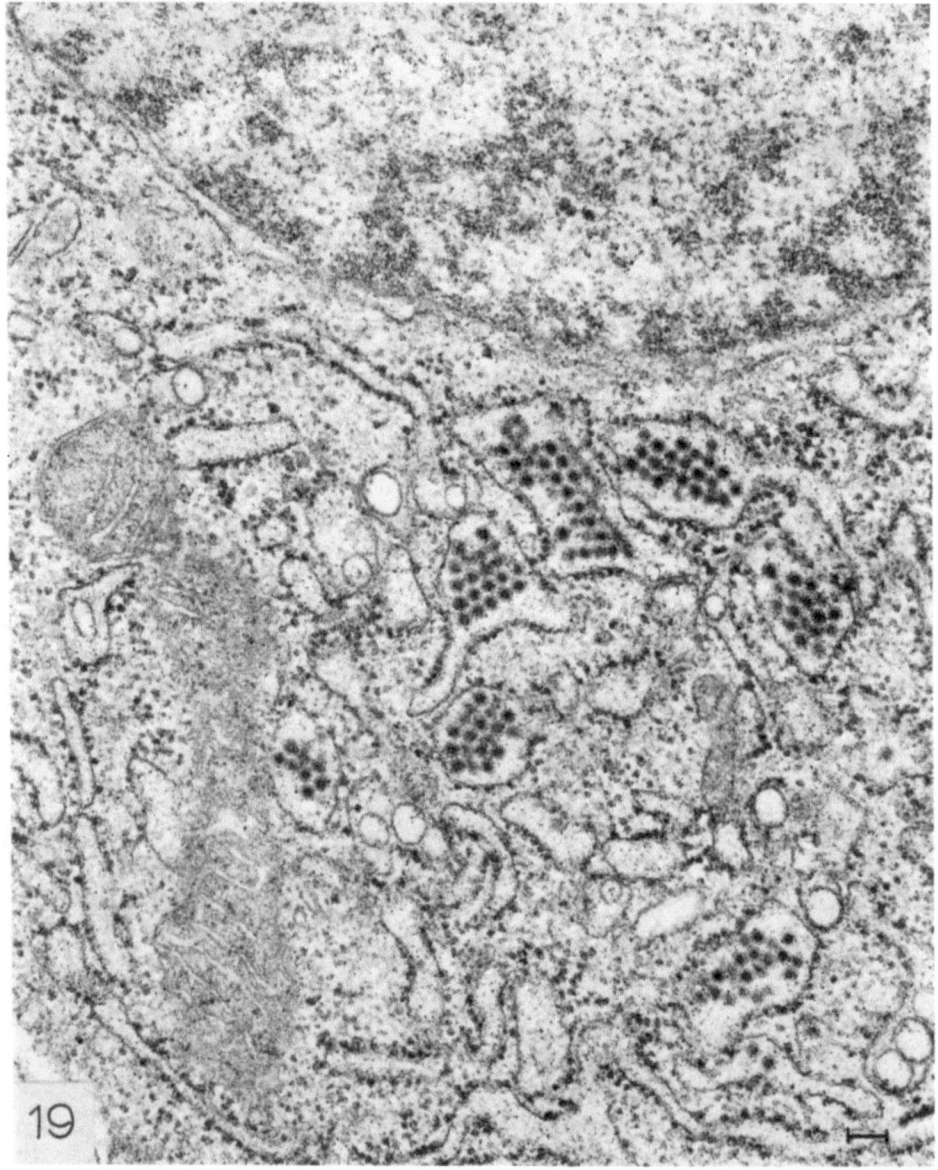

Fig. 19. Crystalline aggregates of virions in cytoplasmic vacuoles of Vero cells 24 hours
after infection with dengue-2 virus. Bar = 100 nm

membrane-enclosed structures (*e.g.*, Golgi apparatus, endoplasmic reticulum) or
to the laying down, *de novo*, of cellular or virus-modified membranes. Some of the
vesicles contain virions which are of "normal" appearance in cross section. Other
viral particles accumulate in sizeable crystalline aggregates in the cytoplasm in a
form suggesting either that they are bound by a membrane or that they arise in
an amorphous matrix (Figs. 19 and 20). No clear evidence has been obtained for

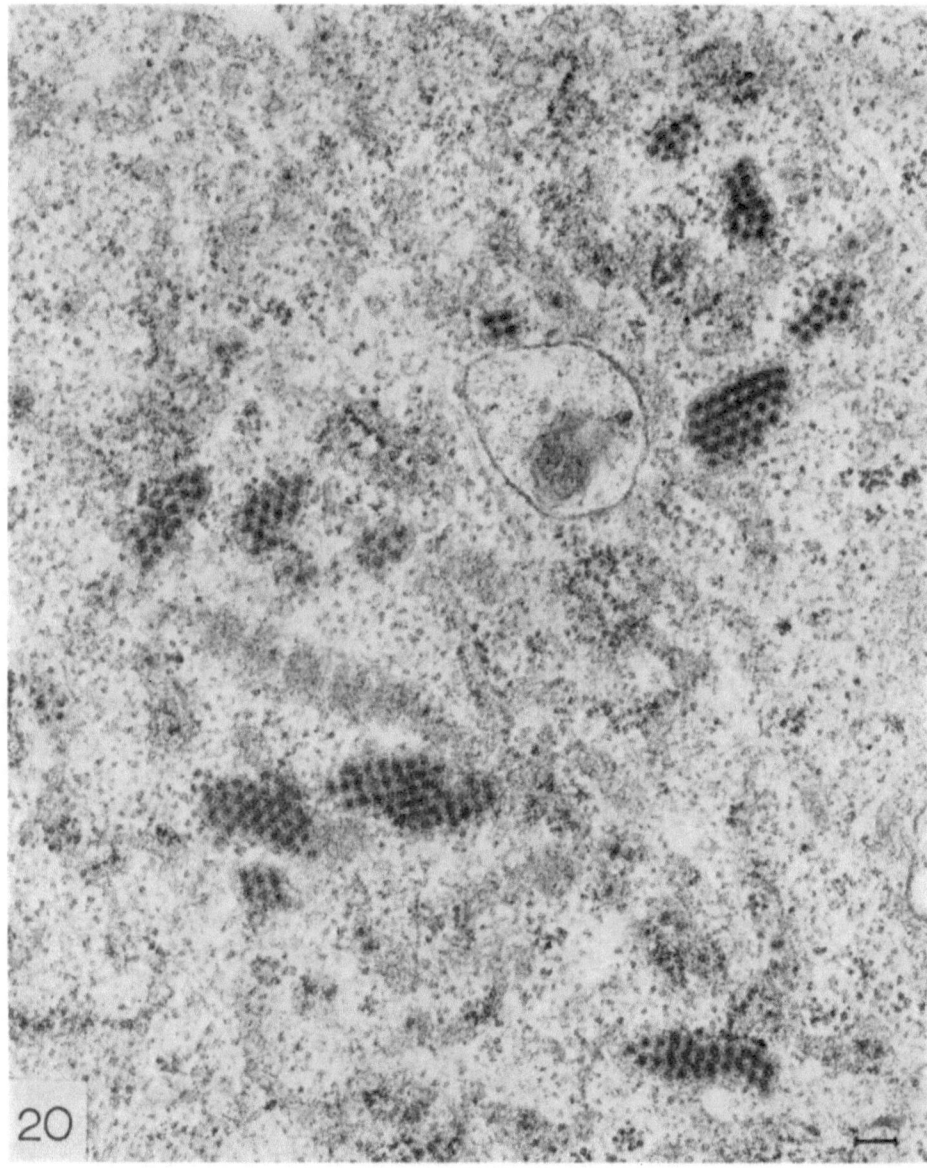

Fig. 20. Crystalline viral aggregates in cytoplasm of Vero cell 36 hours after infection
with dengue-2 virus. No clear evidence for limiting membrane. Bar = 100 nm.
(See also MATSUMURA *et al.*, 1971)

the maturation of these intravesicular or crystalloid virions by a process of budding at a membrane (MATSUMURA *et al.*, 1971; CARDIFF *et al.*, 1973; CATANZARO *et al.*, 1974; DEMSEY *et al.*, 1974; cf. BOULTON and WESTAWAY, 1976). Although the membranes lining virion-containing vacuoles are often studded on the cyto-

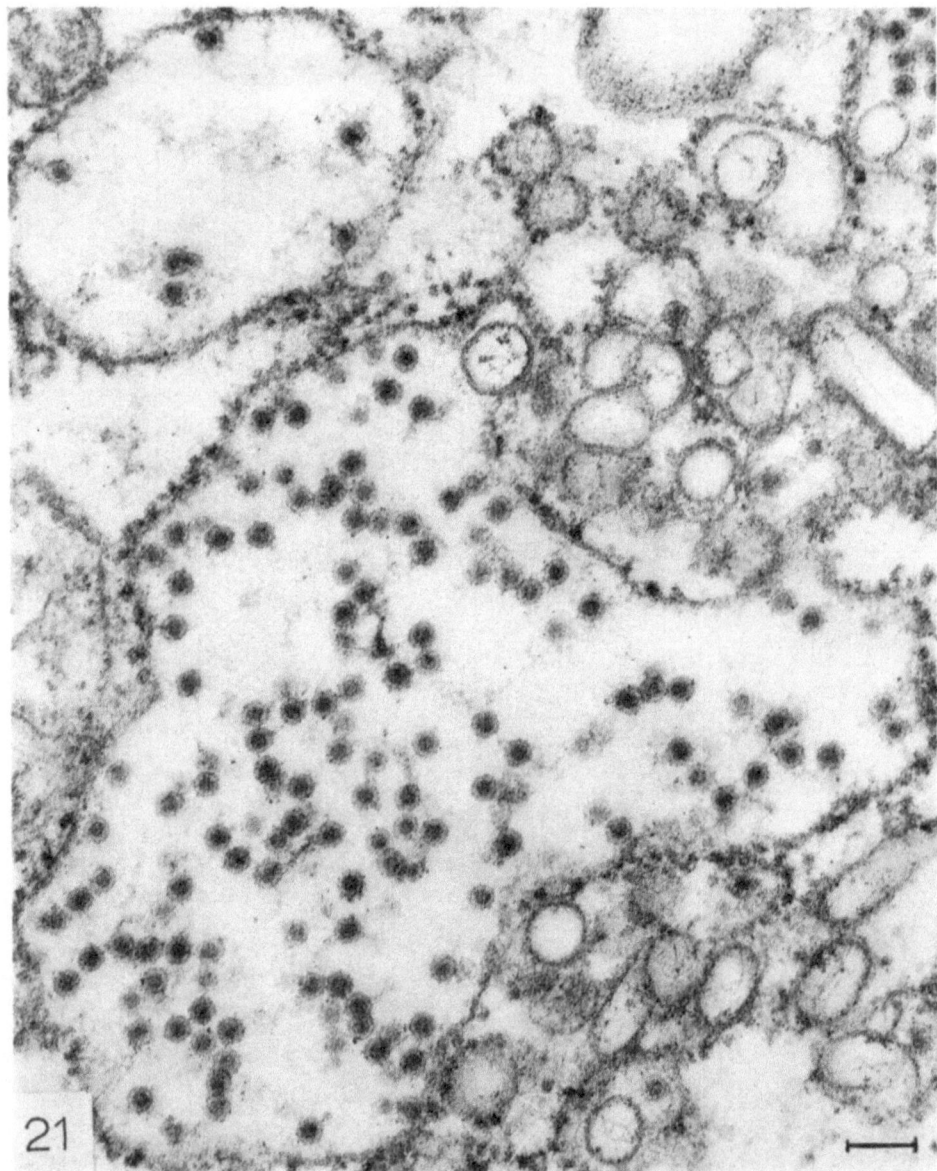

Fig. 21. Large virion-containing cytoplasmic vacuole in Vero cell 24 hours after infection with dengue-2 virus, again showing electron-dense bodies on the cytoplasmic side of the membrane (see also Fig. 6). Bar = 100 nm. From MATSUMURA *et al.* (1971). With permission from Academic Press, Inc., New York

plasmic side with electron-dense bodies measuring 20—30 nm in diameter (Fig. 21), *i.e.*, the probable size of nucleocapsids, their nature has not been identified.

These electron microscopic findings have been correlated by CARDIFF *et al.* (1973) with immunofluorescent localization of dengue 2-specific structural (RHA) and non-structural (SCF) antigens in LLC-MK 2 cells. Toward the end of the latent period, both antigens are demonstrable in the perinuclear region. Eventually, SCF remains in that location, while the structural antigen forms a granular fluorescence throughout the cytoplasm.

In contrast to the situation for group A togaviruses (cf. PFEFFERKORN and SHAPIRO, 1974, for review) the plasma membrane does not seem to be prominently involved in the maturation and release of dengue (or other group B) viruses. It has, however, been demonstrated, through use of peroxidase-labeled antibody, that dengue virus-specific antigen appears on the cell surface at some time between 20 and 36 hours after infection and accumulates thereafter (CATANZARO *et al.*, 1974). At about the same time, the cells also become susceptible to complement-mediated lysis by specific antiviral antibody as measured by ^{51}Cr release (BRANDT and RUSSELL, 1975; CATANZARO *et al.*, 1975). Further consideration of the involvement of cellular membranes in viral morphogenesis will be presented below (Section VII. A. 6.).

b) Effects on Cellular Metabolism

Again in contrast to the group A togaviruses (cf. PFEFFERKORN and SHAPIRO, 1974, for review) which turn off cellular protein synthesis in vertebrate cells rapidly and efficiently, dengue and other group B viruses seem to have a much less pronounced effect. WESTAWAY (1973) has reported that dengue-2-specified protein synthesis in actinomycin D-treated cultures represents roughly 40—50% of total ^{3}H-leucine incorporation in Vero or PS (porcine) cell cultures, even late after infection. The inference that 50—60% of ongoing protein synthesis is cellular *and* that this synthesis continues in infected cells requires critical demonstration that all cells are in fact producing virus.

The only other reference to studies on cellular synthetic processes in group B-infected cells concerns a report by ZEBOVITZ *et al.* (quoted from PFEFFERKORN and SHAPIRO, 1974), to the effect that infection with Japanese encephalitis virus stimulates the synthesis of phospholipids. It is suggested that this response may reflect the proliferation of perinuclear membranous structures, for short pulses of ^{3}H-choline label perinuclear membranes to a greater extent than cytoplasmic membranes.

3. Effects of Metabolic Inhibitors

a) Inhibition of RNA Synthesis

The replication of dengue-2 virus in KB cells is not inhibited by actinomycin D at concentrations of <0.1 µg/ml medium. At higher concentrations, KB cells are visibly damaged. In the range of 0.01—0.03 µg/ml, the yield of virus may be increased slightly over untreated control yields, a finding also reported for Chikungunya virus, a group A togavirus, and attributed to drug-induced inhibition of interferon synthesis (HELLER, 1963). In sister cultures infected with type 2 adenovirus, the yields of this virus were inhibited at actinomycin D concentrations

100-fold below the cytotoxic range, *i.e.*. well within the range at which synthesis of dengue-2 virus was not affected (STOLLAR *et al.*, 1966).

It should be noted that inhibition by actinomycin D of another group B togavirus (Japanese encephalitis) in porcine kidney cell cultures has been reported (ZEBOVITZ *et al.*, 1972) and that a preliminary report has claimed sensitivity of St. Louis encephalitis virus to actinomycin D *early* in the replicative cycle (BRAWNER *et al.*, 1973). These findings as well as some morphological observations have been used as arguments in favor of nuclear involvement in early group B togavirus replication. Further stringent documentation will be required before the evidence can be accepted.

The uridine analogs *5-fluorouridine* and *6-azauridine* (Fig. 17) prevent virus replication at concentrations well below the cytotoxic range. Moreover, as shown in Fig. 22, the formation or release of PFU and HA is inhibited in parallel by 6-azauridine as a function of drug concentration (STOLLAR *et al.*, 1966).

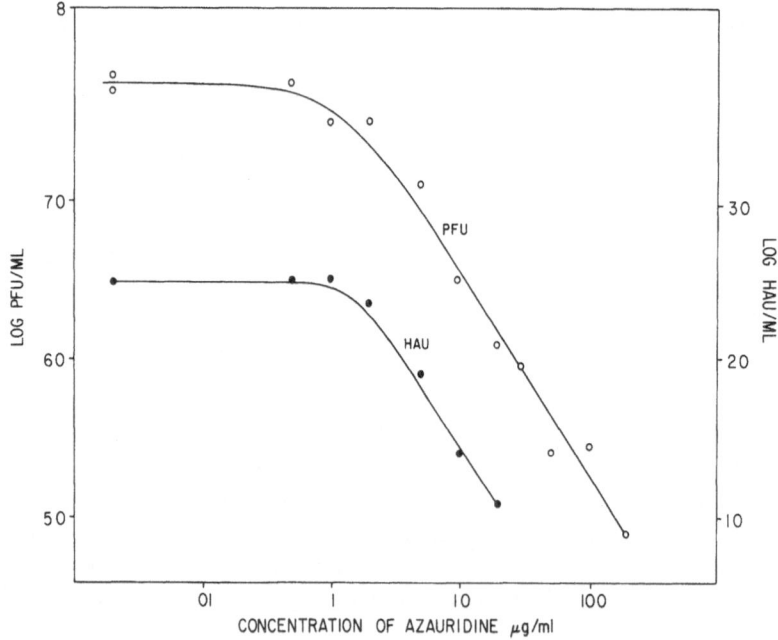

Fig. 22. Dengue-2 virus: Yield (PFU and HAU) from KB cell monolayers as a function of concentration of 6-azauridine.

The drug, at the concentrations indicated, was added to replicate infected cultures immediately after virus adsorption. Forty-eight hours after infection, medium was harvested from each culture and assayed. Modified from STOLLAR *et al.* (1966)

Finally, *guanidine-HCL*, a powerful inhibitor of the replication of certain picornaviruses acting by blocking RNA synthesis, fails to affect dengue-2 virus replication except at concentrations visibly toxic to the cells (Table 14) (STOLLAR, unpublished data).

Table 14. *Effect of guanidine-HCl on growth of dengue-2 virus in KB cells: virus harvested at 24 hours*

Concentration of Guanidine	CPE at 24 hours[a]	Virus yields 24 hours p.i.	
		HAU/ml	PFU/ml
1×10^{-2} M	1—2+	4	1.4×10^6
8×10^{-3} M	2+	25	3.3×10^6
5×10^{-3} M	2+	30	5.0×10^7
2×10^{-3} M	1+	40	1.5×10^7
1×10^{-3} M	1+	80	2.7×10^7
5×10^{-4} M	0—1	60	2.9×10^7
2×10^{-4} M	0—1	80	2.9×10^7
1×10^{-4} M	0	80	3.1×10^7
5×10^{-5} M	0	60	3.8×10^7
2×10^{-5} M	0	60	3.8×10^7
1×10^{-5} M	0	60	3.6×10^7
0	0	60	3.7×10^7

[a] CPE due to toxicity of drug is correlated with reduced virus yields at concentrations above 1×10^{-3} M.

V. STOLLAR, unpublished data.

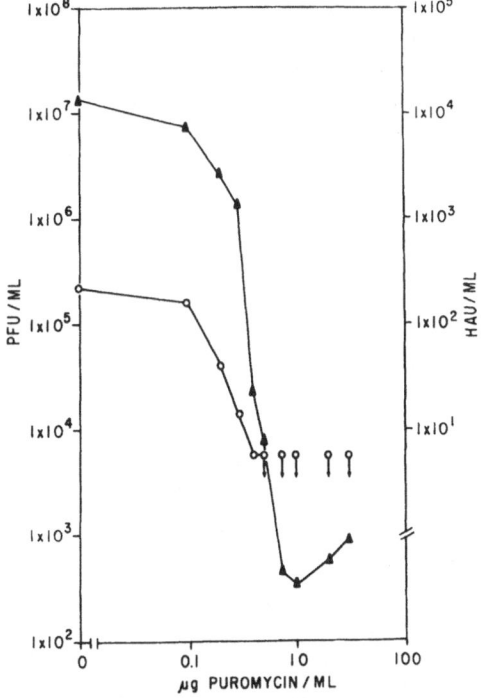

Fig. 23. Dengue-2 virus: Yield (PFU and HAU) from KB cell monolayers as a function of concentration of puromycin. Procedure as in Fig. 22. V. STOLLAR, unpublished data

b) Inhibition of Protein Synthesis

The effect of puromycin is illustrated in Fig. 23, again demonstrating the close parallelism of the dose response in terms of PFU and HA production. Puromycin inhibits virus maturation completely when added up to about 6 hours after infection. Addition between 6 and 24 hours p.i. leads to progressively reduced inhibition. The data suggest that viral RNA (cf. Fig. 17) and protein syntheses occur in parallel and at the same time and are therefore presumably closely coupled (STOLLAR, unpublished data).

4. Viral RNA Replication

a) Rate

As indicated above, the total yield of dengue-2 virus from KB cell cultures is relatively low, and the use of analytical methods and isotope labeling has thus far not permitted the direct determination of the onset and rate of viral RNA synthesis.

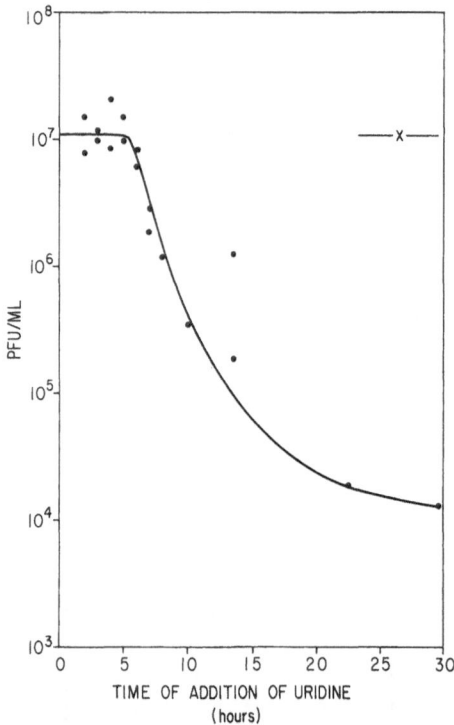

Fig. 24. Yield of dengue-2 virus from KB cell cultures as a function of the time of reversal of 6-azauridine inhibition.

After adsorption, infected cultures were refed with medium containing 6-azauridine (final concentration 15 μg/ml; see Fig. 22). At the times indicated, uridine was added (final concentration 45 μg/ml). At 29 hours after infection, medium was harvested from each treated culture and titrated for PFU. (—×—) Control virus yield at 29 hours in absence of 6-azauridine or uridine. Modified from STOLLAR et al. (1966)

However, these parameters can be estimated indirectly, *i.e.*, by the use of metabolic inhibitors such as 6-azauridine (STOLLAR *et al.*, 1966). The experiments depicted in Figs. 17 and 24 clearly indicate that (a) virus replication begins to become insensitive to 6-azaU inhibition at 6—7 hours after infection, (b) the rate at which this insensitivity develops runs parallel to and precedes virus maturation by about 6 hours (Fig. 17), (c) uridine can reverse the inhibition completely when added at or before 6 hours after infection but reversibility decreases progressively at later times (Fig. 24). These findings suggest that viral RNA synthesis begins about 6 hours after infection and 6 hours prior to viral maturation, and that its rate directly determines the rate at which viral progeny is produced. The fact that the release of HA activity is inhibited by 6-azaU to the same extent as that of infectious virus (see above, Fig. 22) suggests that the production or release of "incomplete" virus (or SHA) particles (see Section VI. A. 2.), which do not contain viral RNA, is also dependent on uninterrupted RNA synthesis or coupled with the maturation and release of infectious virus (see below).

b) Mechanism of RNA Replication

As discussed in Section VI, the genome of dengue-2 virus is a single-stranded RNA molecule of sedimentation coefficient $\sim$45 S and estimated molecular weight 4.2×10^6 daltons. The fact that replication is not inhibited by actinomycin D has made it possible to study viral RNA synthesis under conditions blocking incorporation of labeled precursors into cellular RNA. The sedimentation pattern in sucrose gradients of RNA isolated from actinomycin D-treated, dengue-2 infected KB cells is shown in Fig. 25. Major peaks of RNA are found at about 45 and 20 S. Of these, the 45 S species is entirely sensitive to degradation by ribonuclease and has a base composition closely similar to that of mature virion RNA (STOLLAR *et al.*, 1967). The 20 S species is RNase-resistant.

In contrast to the group A togaviruses for which a variety of intracellular single-stranded species and replicative intermediate as well as double-stranded forms have been described (cf. PFEFFERKORN and SHAPIRO, 1974, for summary), the dengue and other group B togaviruses seem to present a somewhat simpler or more elusive picture.

First, and in contrast to mutually contradictory claims for other group B viruses, STOLLAR *et al.* (1966) were unable to detect in dengue-2 infected KB cells anything unequivocally analogous to the "interjacent" 26 S single-stranded RNA so prominent in group A-infected cells.

Secondly, the fact that the 20 S replicative form (RF), upon denaturation with dimethyl sulfoxide (DMSO) (KATZ and PENMAN, 1966) is converted, with an efficiency of about 95%, to a form sedimenting at about 45 S and no other double-stranded forms are encountered consistently (STOLLAR *et al.*, 1967) suggests that the viral RNA is replicated as a single base-paired linear molecule. Short pulse labeling experiments which might reveal heterodisperse replicative intermediate forms have not yet been done.

Thirdly, base analysis of 20 S RF labeled with ^{32}P at different times after infection has revealed that both strands are synthesized only in the early (latent) phase of infection while after 12 hours only the virion (+) strand is made (STOLLAR *et al.*, 1967). This sequence of events, taken together with the infectiousness of virion RNA, tells us (1) that the latter is of "plus" (messenger) polarity, (2) that, presumably, parental RNA is transcribed in its entirety. and (3) that subsequent production of progeny strands again appears to involve uninterrupted transcription of the "minus" template.

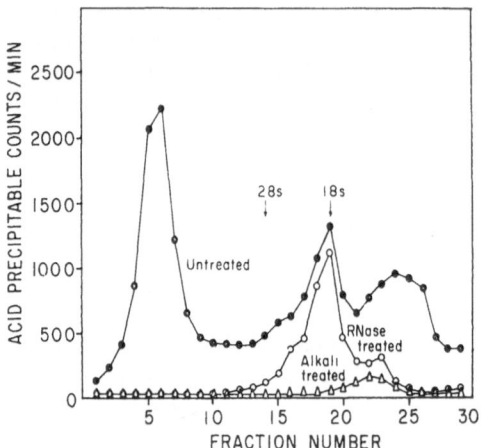

Fig. 25. Ribonuclease treatment of virus-specific RNA from infected cells.
KB cells in 75 cm² flasks (each containing 1.2×10^7 cells) were infected with dengue-2 virus. Twenty-three hours after infection, actinomycin D (final concentration 3 μg/ml) was added, and after one more hour, uridine-³H (specific activity 17.3 Ci/mmole) to a final concentration of 12 μCi/ml. After 2 hours of exposure to the uridine-³H, the cells were harvested. The RNA was extracted at 20° with 10^{-3} M potassium phosphate, pH 7.4, replacing sodium acetate in the extraction medium. RNA was then centrifuged through a 5—20% sucrose gradient and 1 ml fractions were collected. Three 0.15 ml portions were taken from each fraction, for determination of acid-precipitable radioactivity after (1) no further treatment, (2) incubation with RNase (final concentration 2 μg/ml, 12 minutes 37°), (3) incubation in 0.3 N KOH for 16 hours at 37°. Arrows indicate position of optical density peaks due to ribosomal RNA. From STOLLAR *et al.* (1967)
With permission of the authors and Academic Press, Inc., New York

Except for the failure thus far to demonstrate heterodisperse replicative intermediates, the most straightforward model of dengue viral RNA replication would be patterned after that generally accepted for picornavirus RNA (cf. BALTIMORE, 1971). This model would imply either (1) that the parental and progeny strands function as polycistronic mRNA or (2) that secondary processing of the transcription product occurs prior to association with polyribosomes. Alternative (1) would require either primary translation into a single precursor protein with subsequent cleavage (as in the picorna systems) or regulated initiation and termination at multiple sites. Alternative (2) would require post-transcriptional cleavage yielding multiple species of polysome-associated polyadenylated RNA of <45S. No virus-specific polyribosomes have thus far been isolated from cells infected with dengue or other group B togaviruses. This is clearly one of the major holes in our current knowledge about these viruses. Evidence regarding alternative (1) is discussed in the next section.

A single report describing the activity of an apparently dengue-2 induced RNA polymerase suggests that the reaction product is heterodisperse RNase-sensitive RNA, peaking at ~26S (CARDIFF et al., 1973a). This enzyme activity has so far been measured only in crude LLC-MK2 cell extracts ("mitochondrial fraction"). In this form, it is apparently membrane-bound and requires Mg^{++}. Further work is needed to clarify the nature of this polymerase and of its product(s).

5. Synthesis of Virus-Specific Proteins

Polypeptide analyses of cells infected with dengue-2 and various other group B togaviruses (SHAPIRO et al., 1972b, c; TRENT and QURESHI, 1971; QURESHI and TRENT, 1973a; WESTAWAY, 1973, 1975) have revealed a remarkably consistent pattern summarized in Table 15 (from WESTAWAY, 1973); four major and three less well resolved non-virion polypeptides (NV-5, -4, -2, -1 and NV-3, -X, and 2½, respectively), together with the virion polypeptide V-3 and -2 (Figs. 12—14). Of these, NV-2, V-3, and NV-3 are glycosylated. Thus far, no definitive role has been assigned to any of the nonstructural (NV) proteins. Coincidence of PAGE migration rates of the type-specific cell-associated "Antigen III" of QURESHI and TRENT (1973a) with NV-5 ("NSP-1" in the earlier terminology of these authors) suggests a relationship, but no functional role for either has been suggested. In particular, there are no data clearly identifying any one protein as a precursor of another one. NV-2 has been suggested as a possible precursor for V-1, as discussed more fully in the following Section (VII. A. 6.).

It was shown by SHAPIRO et al. (1972c) that, in the case of JE virus, all cell-associated virus-specified proteins are mainly membrane-bound and not detectable in soluble form in cytoplasmic extract. Subsequently, the same group reported presence of all viral polypeptides in smooth and rough membrane fractions (KOS et al., 1975). This was confirmed in a more detailed study by STOHLMAN et al. (1975) for dengue type 2-infected BHK-21 cells: these authors concluded that viral RNA as well as protein synthesis was localized on the rough endoplasmic reticulum but that glycosylation occurred mainly in the smooth membranes and those intermediate between smooth and rough. Relatively low levels of nucleocapsid protein VP-2 led them to postulate that the same membrane fraction was the probable site for virion maturation and release.

Finally, an extensive paper by BOULTON and WESTAWAY (1976), describing similar work on Kunjin virus in Vero cells, appeared just as this manuscript was in final revision. They report somewhat better resolution of the various membrane fractions. In particular, their conclusion is that RNA synthesis occurs predominantly on smooth membranes, protein synthesis on rough membranes. While PAGE profiles of proteins are similar on all membrane fractions, glycosylation patterns show some differences in the rates of incorporation of specific sugars in the various fractions. Envelope glycoprotein VP-3 is deficient in glucosamine in the smooth membrane fraction. Of special interest may be the finding that all viral proteins are rapidly transferred to the plasma membrane and that the largest nonstructural protein, NV-5, shows enrichment in the plasma membrane.

The following additional points are noteworthy about the cell membrane-associated polypeptides: (a) the absence of virion polypeptide V-1; (b) absence

Table 15. *Molecular weights of virion (V) and of nonvirion (NV) proteins specified by group B togaviruses (daltons $\times 10^{-3}$)*

Virus-cell system	NV-5	NV-4	Envelope protein V-3	NV-3	NV-X	NV-2½	NV-2	Core protein V-2	NV-1	Virion protein V-1	Source of data
Kunjin Vero and PS	98[a]	70.5	51.3	44	32	21	19	13.5	10.3	8.5[b]	WESTAWAY (1973)
Japanese encephalitis Vero and PS	96.5	69	53	46	31	21	19	13.7	10.3	Abs.[b]	WESTAWAY (1973)
Chick	93	71	53	45	[c]	.	19	13.5	10.5	8.7	SHAPIRO et al. (1971)
Dengue type 2 Vero and PS	98	75	59	49	34	21	17.7	13.5	9	Abs.	WESTAWAY (1973)
BHK21	92	75	59	48.5	—	—	19	15.5	9	7.0	STOHLMAN et al. (1975)
KB (virions)	—	—	59	—	—	—	19	13.5	.	7.7	STOLLAR (1969)
St. Louis encephalitis Vero and PS	98	70.5	51.3	44	32	21	19	13.5	10.3	Abs.	WESTAWAY (1973)
BHK (virions)	—	—	63	—	—	—	—	18	—	8.5	TRENT and QURESHI (1971)
Sindbis virions Vero (as markers)	—	—	53	—	—	—	—	30	—	—	WESTAWAY (1973)

[a] Molecular weights were calculated after co-electrophoresis of group B virus proteins labeled in infected cytoplasm of Vero cells and of PS cells with Sindbis envelope and core proteins as markers on 8% SDS phosphate polyacrylamide gels. The estimates were verified by then using the Kunjin virus proteins (with their derived molecular weights) also as markers in co-electrophoresis with the other group B togaviruses. Only some of the electrophoretic profiles are shown in the quoted figures.

[b] V-1 is absent from electrophoretic profiles of infected cytoplasm; it remains in cores derived from virions by deoxycholate treatment but not after treatment with a nonionic detergent (references: WESTAWAY and REEDMAN, 1969; SHAPIRO et al. (1971); STOLLAR (1969); TRENT and QURESHI (1971).

[c] A dash indicates that no molecular weight estimate for this protein is available from the quoted reference.

Modified from WESTAWAY (1973).

of a polypeptide peak corresponding to the soluble CF antigen (SCF), MW 39,000 daltons, isolated from dengue-infected mouse brain or cell cultures; (c) an aggregate molecular weight for all virus-specified proteins of about 380,000 daltons, *i.e.*, satisfying at least 75 per cent of the coding capacity of a genome of 4.2×10^6 daltons; (d) absence of a giant polypeptide that could be a candidate for a primary translational precursor.

In keeping with the last point, WESTAWAY (1973) employed short pulse-long chase as well as amino acid analog experiments to observe posttranslational cleavage in Kunjin virus-infected Vero or BHK-21 cells. He was unable to demonstrate it. Instead he found all proteins except the nucleocapsid polypeptide VP-2 to be remarkably stable.

It should be noted that these methods were not entirely successful in the search for precursor proteins in group A virus infection either, and that more conclusive results in that case came from studies of temperature-sensitive (ts) mutants and from use of specific tryptic enzyme inhibitors (reviewed by PFEFFER-KORN and SHAPIRO, 1974). No comparable work has as yet been reported for the group B togaviruses.

6. Viral Morphogenesis

a) Current Ideas and Possible Alternatives

As has been indicated, electron microscopic studies have brought to light quantitative differences between dengue-infected human or hamster cells on one hand and monkey kidney cells on the other. The former generally reveal less striking CPE and accumulation of virus particles than Vero and LLC-MK2 cells (MATSUMURA et al., 1971). In the latter, virus replication is associated with prominent proliferation of membrane-bound vacuoles and the appearance of crystalline aggregates of virion-like particles in the cytoplasm (cf. Figs. 19—21, above).

This quantitative contrast is paradoxical because the yield of extracellular infectious dengue-2 virus from KB cells is at least equivalent to or higher than that from monkey cells. Yet, these observations form the basis for the claim that dengue and other group B viruses, in contrast to group A togaviruses, mature and are released in association with internal cytoplasmic membranes rather than the outer plasma membrane. The fact is that none of the cell systems thus far examined have furnished convincing morphological support for the release of virions by budding from any membranes While this lack of visualization may be simply a consequence of inadequate levels or rates of virus production, one should not exclude the following alternate possibilities.

Alternative (a): *The viral envelope is not derived from defined preformed cellular membranes* (analogous to group A and other enveloped viruses) *but is laid down, de novo, in a cytoplasmic matrix* (*i.e.*, analogous to the cytoplasmic "factories" in poxvirus replication). Evidence for this possibility is the appearance of crystalline viral aggregates in the cytoplasm of monkey kidney cells (cf. Figs. 19, 20). One *could* view the virus-filled vacuoles (MATSUMURA et al., 1971; CARDIFF et al., 1973 b; CATANZARO et al., 1974; DEMSEY et al., 1974; STOHLMAN et al., 1975) as a secondary sequestration of such "factories".

Alternative (b): *Maturation and release of infectious virions does, after all, occur at the plasma membrane, not at intracytoplasmic membranes.* Evidence for this is (i) relatively modest cytoplasmic accumulation in a relatively productive (KB) cell species, (ii) demonstration of viral antigen at the cell surface (CATANZARO et al., 1974), (iii) association of structural and nonstructural viral proteins and glycoproteins with plasma membrane as well as other membrane fractions of infected cells (STOHLMAN et al., 1975; BOULTON and WESTAWAY, 1976), (iv) the rapid and pronounced effect of changes in medium composition on the nature of the virus that is released (see below). (v) features of viral replication in cultured mosquito cells (see Section VII. B.).

Alternative (c): Combining (a) and (b); *the formation of virus-filled cytoplasmic aggregates and vacuoles is characteristic of cells in which the normal maturation and release mechanism via plasma membrane is inefficient, i.e., they are the dead end of an aborted process of virion assembly.* Evidence favoring this view is the unexpectedly low yield of infectious virus obtained from Vero or LLC-MK 2 (MATSUMURA et al., 1971) cell cultures containing vast numbers of virions in each cell (cf. Figs. 19, 20) (see further discussion below, Section VII. C.). Moreover, the distribution of all viral polypeptides except VP-1 in all membranes could also be interpreted as favoring this view.

Current knowledge does not permit a decision among these alternatives. including the generally preferred one invoking release from cytoplasmic membranes followed by disgorgement of aggregated virions by transport from vacuoles or "lamellar cisternae" (SRIURAIRATNA et al., 1973; BOULTON and WESTAWAY. 1976) to the surface. However, the following facts have a bearing on the problem of morphogenesis and its eventual clarification. Much of the work summarized was done by SHAPIRO and his colleagues on Japanese encephalitis virus but, where examined, dengue-2 virus has shown similar features.

b) Different Forms of Virus-Specific Particles

(1) Extracellular particles consist of (i) infectious hemagglutinating virions ["complete" virus (STEVENS and SCHLESINGER, 1965; STOLLAR. 1969; STOLLAR et al., 1966) or rapidly sedimenting hemagglutinin "RHA" (SMITH et al.. 1970) or "N" forms (SHAPIRO et al., 1972 b)]. These are, as already discussed, characterized by possessing a 45 S viral genome, 3 virion polypeptides (VP-1, -2, -3), and by having a PFU/HA ratio ranging between $10^{4.3}$ and $10^{6.0}$; (ii) noninfectious hemagglutinating particles ["incomplete" virus (STEVENS and SCHLESINGER, 1965; STOLLAR et al., 1966, 1967; STOLLAR, 1969) or slowly sedimenting HA ("SHA") subviral particles (SMITH et al., 1970; CARDIFF et al., 1971)]. These are particles lacking 45 S RNA (STOLLAR et al., 1966) and the capsid protein V-2 (STOLLAR 1969; SHAPIRO et al., 1971) and possessing variable proportions of VP-1 or the non-virion protein NV-2 (SHAPIRO et al., 1971; CARDIFF et al., 1971; see below). They are believed to represent excess envelope material which is released along with complete virions.

(2) Intracellular ("I" or cell-associated) particles have sedimentation characteristics similar to those of normal virions. They appear to be of "normal" morphology (cf. Figs. 6, 21) in that they possess an electron dense core and an envelope. They are presumed to contain 45 S viral RNA but lack virion polypeptide VP-1 which is replaced by non-virion glycopolypeptide NV-2 (SHAPIRO et al.. 1972 b, 1973 a). These "I" forms have been reported to contain a higher ratio of

envelope proteins (VP-3 + NV-2) to nucleocapsid protein (VP-2) than do "N" forms [(VP-3 + VP-1)/VP-2] (cf. PFEFFERKORN and SHAPIRO, 1974). Cell-associated virus, presumably representing the "I"-form of SHAPIRO et al. (1972b; 1973b), displays relatively low infectivity (MATSUMURA et al., 1972). No conclusive information regarding HA activity of cell-associated dengue-2 virus is available; preliminary experiments by CLEAVES and MARCHETTA in our laboratory have suggested its presence after treatment of cell extracts with polyethylene glycol and protamine, but it is impossible to judge at this time whether the HA represents aggregated cytoplasmic virions or particles in process of maturation and release. It should be remembered, however, that rigorous criteria for calculating the specific biological activity of dengue virions in terms of particle/PFU/HAU ratios are lacking (see below).

(3) Experimental modification of virus release. When infected cells are incubated in TRIS-containing medium rather than in standard medium, *"T"-form virions* are released which resemble "I" virions in relatively low infectivity and replacement of V-1 by NV-2 (SHAPIRO et al., 1972b; 1973a).

These observations have led SHAPIRO et al. (1972b) to postulate that the maturation of dengue and other group B viruses occurs in association with cytoplasmic membranes or vacuoles and that it involves the cleavage of virus-specified intra-

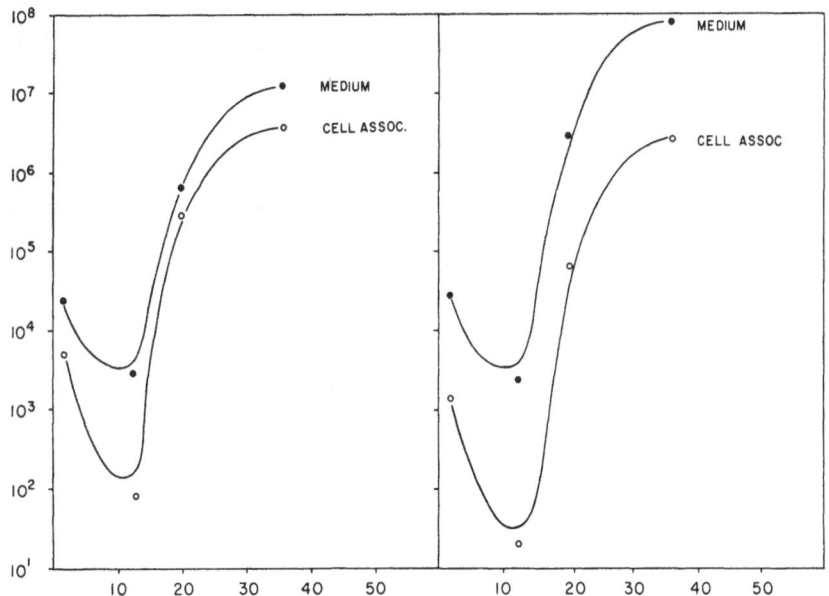

Fig. 26. Effect of MgSO$_4$ on the yield of extracellular (•—•) and cell-associated (o—o) dengue-2 virus.
Vero cells were infected with dengue virus and maintained in the usual manner. After the 12 hours samples were taken, MgSO$_4$ was added to one set of cultures (final concentration 33 mM), and a similar volume of isotonic phosphate buffered saline to another set. At the time indicated, media and cells were harvested for assay of extracellular and cell-associated virus. Left panel: Control cultures. Right panel: MgSO$_4$ added. From MATSUMURA et al. (1972a)
With permission of the authors and Cambridge University Press

cellular membrane glycoprotein NV-2 (MW 18,000—19,000 daltons, see Table 15), to yield the non-glycosylated virion envelope protein V-1 (MW 7,700 daltons. see Table 15). They further postulate that this cleavage is inhibited by TRIS and that, therefore, released "T" virions resemble the intracellular "I" form (SHAPIRO *et al.*, 1972b, 1973a). Direct proof for this interesting proposal, *e.g.*, in the form of pulse-chase experiments or of peptide mapping of NV-2 and V-1, is still lacking.

Another experimental procedure that affects the release of dengue virions quantitatively and qualitatively involves variations in ionic strength of the medium. It has been shown by MATSUMURA *et al.* (1972a) that increases in concentration of $MgCl_2$, $MgSO_4$, or NaCl lead to significant increases in infectious titer and that this effect is manifest within 5 minutes or less (MATSUMURA *et al.*, 1972a, b) of the addition of salt. The enhancement is demonstrable *only* in terms of released, *not* of cell-associated virus (Fig. 26). Moreover, high ionic strength promotes the release of HA even more strikingly than that of PFU (Table 16).

Table 16. *Effect of varying concentrations of $MgCl_2$ on the release of dengue-2 virus from Vero cells*

Conc. of $MgCl_2$ from 10—24 hours after infection (mM)	Titers 10 hours p.i. before add'n of $MgCl_2$		Titers 24 hours p.i. 14 hours after add'n of $MgCl_2$		
	PFU/ml	HAU/ml	PFU/ml	HAU/ml	PFU/HAU (log_{10})
1	9.3×10^2	<5	6.3×10^6	10	5.8
10	10.2×10^2	<5	10.4×10^6	10	6.0
20	8.2×10^2	<5	16.1×10^6	20	5.9
30	8.4×10^2	<5	19.6×10^6	40	5.7
40	8.4×10^2	<5	27.1×10^6	80	5.5
50	11.2×10^2	<5	37.0×10^6	160	5.3
60	8.7×10^2	<5	29.4×10^6	320	5.0
80	8.8×10^2	<5	19.3×10^6	160	5.1
100	9.0×10^2	<5	2.0×10^6	20	5.0

Modified from MATSUMURA *et al.* (1972).

This finding suggests that the release of "complete" (RHA or "N") as well as of "incomplete" (SHA or 70S) particles can be influenced by a single experimental manipulation. No analysis of the total yield obtained from high ionic strength cultures has been reported, specifically with regard to separation of "RHA" from "SHA" or to polypeptide patterns. It is tempting, however, to look upon this effect of varying ionic strength as related to the inhibition of Sindbis virus budding and release at low ionic strength (reviewed by PFEFFERKORN and SHAPIRO, 1974) and to suggest that the profundity and rapidity of the enhancement could best be explained in terms of a response of the cell surface rather than of intracellular sites.

B. Mosquito Cells

SINGH and PAUL (1968) first succeeded in maintaining dengue viruses of types 1, 2, 3 and 4 in a mosquito cell line which had been established by SINGH

(1967) from larvae of *Aedes albopictus*, one of the natural vectors of dengue. Although the maximum titers of virus present in the culture fluids were not high (10^2 to 10^3 mouse intracerebral LD_{50}), active virus was detected in the cultures for at least 20 days, suggestive of some continuing viral multiplication. It was noted that strains representing types 1, 2 and 4 exerted cytopathic effects on the cultured cells. A cell line established similarly from larvae of *Aedes aegypti*, another natural dengue vector, did not support growth of the dengue viruses tested in this study.

Subsequent reports from the same laboratory recorded not only the attainment of much higher dengue-2 virus titers in the *A. albopictus* cell line (PAUL and SINGH, 1969) but also significant cytopathic effects induced by all 4 dengue types (PAUL et al., 1969). The latter consisted of cytolysis, syncytium formation, formation of multinucleated giant cells and phagocytosis of affected cells, followed by ultimate recovery of the infected cultures (cf. SINGH, 1971).

High yields of dengue-2 virus in SINGH's *A. albopictus* cell line were reported by SUITOR and PAUL (1969). After infection at a MOI = 5 PFU (assayed on PS-Y 15 cells), the first increase in virus was noted after 5—6 days. These authors also noted the formation of multinucleate cells, ultimately involving the entire cell sheet in one syncytium. This was observed only in cells grown on plastic, not on glass surfaces. Some success in obtaining plaque formation by dengue-1, -2 and -4 viruses in monolayers of SINGH's *A. albopictus* cell line was reported by CORY and YUNKER (1972).

The occurrence or absence of CPE in *A. albopictus* cell cultures after infection with dengue-1 was shown by SWEET and UNTHANK (1971) to be a function of the degree of "adaptation" to the mouse: while human acute phase serum and early mouse passage virus were reported to have $TCID_{50}$ titers in these cells roughly equivalent to the intracerebral mouse LD_{50}, no CPE was observed with virus that had undergone 24 or more mouse passages. In contrast, they reported that various strains of dengue-2 produced marked CPE regardless of their passage level. This was not found by STEVENS (1970) with seed virus of dengue-2 (New Guinea "B" strain) which had undergone 63 passages in mice and 10 passages in human (KB) cell cultures. It should be noted that, while the yield of virus in STEVENS' experiments was low (2×10^4 PFU/ml), the kinetics of viral replication was similar to that in vertebrate cells.

The fact that certain strains of dengue virus, particularly primary isolates, induce significant fusion and syncytium formation in cultures of *Aedes albopictus* cells (PAUL et al., 1969; SUITOR and PAUL, 1969; CHAPPEL et al., 1971) is of special interest. Characteristically, this effect occurs several days after infection and therefore does not represent fusion from without. This finding would strongly imply that a modification of the cellular plasma membrane is associated with virus replication, possibly with maturation and release.

Virus released from *A. albopictus* cells has been reported to be exclusively in the "RHA" fraction, i.e., no "incomplete" or SHA particles are found (SINARACHATA-NANT and OLSON, 1973). This result could be interpreted as reflecting a more efficiently coordinated assembly and release mechanism from these cells than from vertebrate cells. It should be noted, however, that mosquito cell-associated dengue virions have not yet been examined with regard to relative infectiousness and that no polypeptide analysis of either extracellular or intracellular virus has been reported. SINARACHATANANT and OLSON (1973) have also reported that dengue-2 HA derived from mosquito cells is strongly inhibited by antiserum prepared against uninfected mosquito cells while virus grown in LLC-MK2 cells is not inhibited by anti-cell serum against either species. [Similar experiments with Sindbis virus from *A. albopictus* cells (STOLLAR *et al.*, 1975) revealed extremely low-titered HI by anti-cell serum].

HANNOUN and ECHALIER (1971) have reported evidence suggesting some replication, and certainly prolonged persistence, of dengue-1, -2 and -3 viruses in an established diploid line of *Drosophila melanogaster* cells.

Persistent infection of mosquito cell cultures with dengue viruses will be discussed in Section VII. D.

C. Critical Summary Regarding Morphogenesis, Maturation and Release of Dengue Virions

The following points, reviewed above, appear to be reasonably well supported: (i) prominent cytological evidence of infection involves intense cytoplasmic vacuolization, especially in the perinuclear region; (ii) in certain kinds of cells (monkey kidney cell lines, Vero and LLC-MK2) but not in others (human KB and hamster BHK-21), virions are found abundantly in cytoplasmic vacuoles or in (sometimes membrane-bound) crystalline aggregates. Both types of structure seem to contain a matrix of amorphous material; (iii) budding of virions in association with either cytoplasmic or plasma membranes has not been convincingly demonstrated; (iv) there is some evidence suggesting that cytoplasmic vacuoles may be connected by canaliculi to the extracellular environment and that their membranes may fuse with the plasma membranes, perhaps releasing virions in this way (DEMSEY *et al.*, 1974); a system of lamellar cisternae containing chains of single virus particles has been demonstrated in the neurons of dengue-2 infected suckling mouse brains (SRIURAIRATNA *et al.*, 1973) and of Kunjin-infected Vero cells (BOULTON and WESTAWAY, 1976); the possible relationship of such membrane-bound beads of virions to the maturation and release is intriguing; (v) an alternate manner of release proposed is that of "reverse pinocytosis", *i.e.*, the disgorgement of virions from intracellular vacuoles to the outside; (vi) intracellular virions are characterized by low infectiousness and by lack of the virion envelope polypeptide V-1. The latter is replaced by the non-virion glycoprotein NV-2 which is believed to be a precursor of V-1; (vii) extracellular virions are of *relatively* high infectiousness, carry HA activity, and contain the small envelope non-glycosylated protein V-1 which is believed to be a cleavage product of NV-2; (viii) in addition to infectious virions, non-infectious HA material ("incomplete" virus, SHA, 70S HA) is released which lacks 45S viral RNA as well as the *capsid* polypeptide V-2 and contains variable proportions of NV-2 and V-1; (ix) modifications of the medium (*e.g.*, TRIS or ionic strength) can affect the nature of extracellular virus populations; (x) dengue virus replication in cultured mosquito cells may induce cell fusion and syncytium formation; (xi) the virus population released from mosquito cells is apparently more homogeneous than that from vertebrate cells in that the SHA particles are not found.

Although the weight of morphological evidence points to a key role of cytoplasmic membranes and vacuoles in the replication, maturation and release of virus, much of this imagery has been obtained rather late after infection (18 hours being the earliest in an infectious process with a 12 hour latent period); this is true not only for dengue but also for other group B togaviruses. The most active maturation and release of virus occurs between 12 and 36 hours p.i. — yet much of the morphological and biochemical evidence thus far published rests on observations made at 24—48 hours or even later. The question of the *primacy* of cytoplasmic vacuolization and virion aggregation in viral maturation and release requires more rigorous documentation than is now available. It should be recalled that in group A togavirus-infected cells there is also a variable predominance of intracytoplasmic vacuolation or of plasma membrane involvement (cf. PFEFFERKORN and SHAPIRO, 1974). It seems quite possible that a small proportion of the total viral mass produced in cells is, in fact, released from the plasma membrane or at the juncture of cytoplasmic and external membranes and that this minority is what we measure as infectious extracellular yield. The fusion and syncytium formation in infected mosquito cell cultures could be explained on the basis of virus-induced modification of cellular surface (plasma) membranes.

Crucial to this problem is the evaluation of criteria for the total number of virus particles produced and released by a cell. Particle counts have not been reported. One can perhaps derive a rough estimate of the number of physical particles from the HA titer, provided the analogy to influenza virus and Sindbis virus in terms of particle/HAU ratio is valid. For the latter viruses it has been ascertained that the HA titer (*i.e.*, the highest virus dilution which yields a pattern of complete HA) corresponds, within reasonable limits of error, to that virus dilution in which the number of particles is roughly equal to the number of erythrocytes in the HA reaction mixture (WERNER and SCHLESINGER, 1954; DONALD and ISAACS, 1954; STOLLAR et al., 1975). Thus, the total number of particles (N) per ml can be estimated by multiplying the number of RBC (*e.g.*, 10^7) by the reciprocal of the HA titer (H). The product ($H \times 10^7$) would not discriminate between infectious and noninfectious HA particles. If each hemagglutinating particle were also a plaque former, the ratio PFU/N should be 1.0 or, alternatively, the ratio PFU/HAU = 10^7. If only 10% of the total HA particles registered as plaque formers, the latter ratio should be reduced to 10^6, and so on.

In the experimental series depicted in Table 16 (from MATSUMURA et al., 1972a) the PFU/HA ratio varied from 10^5 to 10^6 (in this case as a function of $MgCl_2$ concentration), suggesting that only 1—10% of the HA particles were measurable as plaque formers and that the actual number of physical particles ($H \times 10^7$) *released* ranged from 1×10^8/ml (at 1 mM $MgCl_2$) to 3.2×10^9/ml (at 60 mM $MgCl_2$).

If most of these consist of 14 nm "SHA" particles, they would not be discernible in thin sections since they do not contain viral genomes or nucleocapsid proteins. In terms of infectious virus released, the maximum yields indicated in Fig. 26 are 10^7 to 10^8 PFU per culture or 10—100 virions per cell. Assuming high efficiency of plating, this would represent less than 1 visible virion per 300 Å section of a whole cell. Thus, failure to visualize virus in the process of release is not at all surprising. These considerations lead to the inescapable conclusion that the virus masses seen in the cytoplasm of Vero and LLC-MK 2 cells do not contribute significantly to the infectious virus recovered from the medium of infected cultures but represent an excess, a dead-end accumulation of incompletely processed virions.

D. Persistently Infected Cell Cultures

It was observed by BEASLEY *et al.* (1960) and by SCHULZE (1962) and SCHULZE and SCHLESINGER (1963a) that KB cell monolayer cultures infected with two different strains of dengue-2 virus continued to produce infectious virus for prolonged periods. Such cultures have been maintained for periods of up to three years during which the yield averaged 1 PFU per cell (STEVENS and SCHLESINGER. 1965). The two systems differed in that BEASLEY *et al.* (1960) observed no cytopathic effects, while SCHULZE and SCHLESINGER (1963a) found the persistently infected state to become stabilized after several cycles of cell degeneration and repopulation. The former authors reported failure to "cure" carrier cultures by subcultivation or by exposure to immune serum. They also reported a significantly reduced yield of and retarded cytopathic response to type 1 poliovirus in dengue-2 carrier cultures compared with uninfected KB cells.

Observations similar to those in persistently infected KB cell cultures have also been recorded for rhesus monkey testis (HOTTA and EVANS, 1956a), green monkey kidney (SHIMAZU *et al.*, 1966), human skin (WIEBENGA, 1961a, b), and HeLa cells (MAGUIRE and MILES, 1965). The latter authors attempted, by cloning. to determine the percentage of virus-yielding HeLa cells in such cultures and arrived at an estimate of 3.3 per cent. However, since the cloning efficiency was apparently much reduced from that of uninfected cells (extent of reduction not stated), this estimate may be excessively low. WIEBENGA (1961b), using immuno-fluorescence, estimated that 10—37% of the cells in his chronically infected human skin cells were antigen producers.

As is the case with naturally or experimentally infected *Aedes*, which retain life-long capacity to transmit dengue and other arthropod-borne togaviruses, so it seems to be axiomatic for cell cultures derived from *A. albopictus* or *A. aegypti* to establish a steady-state relationship to these viruses. This type of persistent infection has been studied in much greater detail with Sindbis virus (cf. recent summary by SCHLESINGER, 1975) than with dengue viruses. However, from the studies by BANERJEE and SINGH (1968) and SINARACHATANANT and OLSON (1973) it is clear that flaviviruses and, in the latter's work specifically dengue-2 virus. establish persistent infection. Of great potential importance are the findings (a) that the persistently infected cell cultures can be subcultured indefinitely, (b) that this process may be associated with progressive loss of plaque-producing capacity at 37° C, and (c) that only *complete* virions ("RHA") but no incomplete ("SHA") material seems to be released by either low or high passage infected cultures (SINARACHATANANT and OLSON, 1973). Further characterization of dengue virus isolated from such cultures. as distinct from acutely infected ones. has not yet been reported.

E. Interference and Interferon Production

Interference with unrelated viruses has been observed not only in cells chronically infected with dengue viruses but also during the initial period of virus production following primary infection. This was first reported by BEASLEY *et al.* (1960) for KB cells infected with dengue-2 and superinfected 2 days later with type 1 poliovirus. The final yield of the latter and the rate of cell destruction were reduced. Freshly isolated strains of dengue-1, -2, -4, after 2 passages in baby mice, failed to produce CPE in monkey kidney cell cultures but interfered with type 1 poliovirus (PAUL and BANERJEE, 1965). BANERJEE (1969b) found that, in interference with poliovirus in monkey cell cultures, one interfering dose of dengue virus was equivalent to one LD_{50} or PFU, and that the yield of dengue virus was not reduced by the superinfection.

Table 17. *Interference with VSV plaque production in MCN cell cultures by dengue-2 virus*

LD_{50} equivalent of dengue-2 virus added on day 0	VSV challenge after		
	1 day	3 days	6 days
10^{6a}	0.01^b	0.01	0.05
10^5	0.09	0.15	0.30
10^4	1.30	0.61	0.84
$10^{5.5}$	—	0.10	—
$10^{5.5}$ (UV)^c	—	0.08	—
$10^{5.5}$ (Heated)^d	—	∼0.30	—

[a] No replication of dengue-2 virus was detectable in unchallenged cultures.

[b] $\text{Fraction} = \dfrac{\text{VSV plaques per ml on pretreated plates}}{\text{VSV plaques per ml on control plates}}$.

[c] Dengue-2 virus, at concentration indicated, was irradiated for 3 minutes (36 cm from germicidal lamp). No infectious virus could be detected by injecting mice with irradiated virus.

[d] Dengue-2 virus, at concentration indicated, was heated at 56° C for 20 minutes. No infectious virus could be detected by injecting mice with heated virus.

In all experiments, dengue-2 virus, MB 57 was diluted in $PBS\text{-}Ca_{10}$. Adsorption: 2 hours at room temperature. VSV was diluted in PBS. Adsorption: 1 hour at room temperature. Modified from SCHULZE (1962).

SCHULZE (1962) examined the ability of dengue-2 virus to interfere with plaque production by vesicular stomatitis virus (VSV) on MCN cells [a subline of mouse L cells used by HENLE et al. (1959) for studies of persistent paramyxovirus infections]. A summary of her results is presented in Table 17 to show that (a) interference operates effectively in a cell line in which the interfering (dengue-2) virus undergoes, at best, minimal replication; (b) interfering capacity of dengue-2 virus is retained undiminished after ultraviolet inactivation and partially after heat inactivation. A "challenge virus resistance" (CVR) test was developed by HALSTEAD et al. (1964b), based on the finding that interference with various indicator viruses was induced in several cell lines, optimally in the grivet monkey kidney cell line BS-C-1, by all prototype dengue viruses. Superinfection was at 8 days after the primary dengue infection, and the response was expressed in terms of dengue virus interfering doses (InD_{50}). Subsequently, the evolving resistance of dengue-infected BS-C-1 cells to type 2 poliovirus was correlated with interferon production (RUSSELL et al., 1966a). MAGUIRE and MILES (1965) also found their persistently infected HeLa cells to produce interferon.

Interference among the dengue viruses or between dengue and other flaviviruses in cultured mosquito cells has not yet been studied. Such investigations would probably be quite revealing because (a) earlier reports indicated some interference between dengue and YF viruses (SABIN, 1952a) but none between dengue-2 and Murray Valley encephalitis virus (LAM and MARSHALL, 1968) in intact *A. aegypti*, (b) it appears that mosquito cells do not produce interferon-like substances (STOLLAR and SHENK, 1973), (c) the studies by SINARACHATANANT and OLSON (1973) discussed in preceding sections suggest that *Aedes* cell cultures produce "RHA" but not "SHA". If all of the "RHA" consisted of infectious virions, this would be reminiscent of the preliminary finding by IGARASHI and STOLLAR (1976) that *A. albopictus* cell cultures fail to produce detectable defective-interfering Sindbis virions under conditions which readily generate them in vertebrate cells. Under such conditions interference, if observed, may point directly at some common step in RNA replication.

VIII. Pathogenesis (Experimental Hosts)

A. Monkey

Monkeys are generally susceptible to dengue viruses. A number of species belonging to *Macacus, Cynomolgus, Cercopithecus, Cercocebus, Papio*, etc., can be infected by bites of virus-harboring mosquitoes or by injection of human dengue virus (in the form of patient's blood or serum) by various routes. Hyperpyrexia and leukopenia, usually of slight degrees, are noted. Viremia occurs about a week after the inoculation of virus, and this may be significant for the maintenance of dengue in nature, forming a possible cycle of monkey-mosquito-monkey transmission. Earlier work on these aspects is covered in articles by BLANC et al. (1929), BLANC and CAMINOPETROS (1930), SIMMONS et al. (1931) and FINDLAY (1932). The results were confirmed and extended by later investigations (TANIGUCHI et al., 1943, 1951; OTAWARA et al., 1943; OGATA and HASHIMOTO, 1944b; SABIN and THEILER, 1944; MISAO et al., 1946a, b; REUL and ERRAERTS, 1949). In some monkeys infected with human dengue virus mild myocarditis or nephritis were noted (TANIGUCHI et al., 1943; 1951; MISAO et al., 1946b).

An apparent infection with low-grade fever, followed by production of specific neutralizing antibody, is obtained in chimpanzees after subcutaneous or intracutaneous injection of human dengue virus (PAUL et al., 1948). New world monkeys (belonging to *Cebus, Ateles, Alouatta, Marikina, Saimiri, Aotus*, etc.) react to dengue virus with antibody production, with or without viremia (ROSEN, 1958).

SWEET et al. (1969) reported that juvenile African green monkeys *(Cercopithecus aethiops)* could be infected with type 1 human dengue virus (in the form of acute phase patient's serum) *orally*. No abnormal clinical or hematological signs were noted, nor was there definite evidence for viremia or oral excretion of virus. The serological responses following oral inoculation were almost equal to, if not better than, those following intracutaneous inoculation. It appeared that the human dengue virus behaved in this species of primate differently from mouse-adapted strains.

Of special interest is a change which strains of dengue virus undergo as a result of continuing intracerebral passages in mice, which manifests itself in increasing neurovirulence for *rhesus* monkeys (SABIN, 1950, 1955). Intracerebral injection of *human* virus produced in monkeys an inapparent infection with focal infiltrative lesions in the brain stem and spinal cord, followed by antibody formation. In contrast, type 1 (Hawaii) virus, after 118 passages in mice, induced paralytic disease "which clinically and histologically was not readily distinguishable from that of poliomyelitis" (SABIN, 1955). NATHANSON *et al.* (1965, 1966, 1967) provided a corollary to these observations in quantitative evaluations of the lesions produced in the central nervous system of monkeys inoculated with various group B arboviruses, including dengue-4. The latter had been propagated through 74 passages in HeLa cell cultures and 2 passages in suckling mice and produced only "extreme weakness" in one of 4 monkeys inoculated intracerebrally. The lesions seen in these animals were minimal and resembled those induced by *attenuated* type 3 poliovirus. For further discussion of these aspects see Section IX on Variation.

More recent studies on immunological responses of monkeys, especially as they relate to sequential infection with dengue and other flaviviruses, will be discussed under Immunization (Section XI).

B. Mouse

The mouse can be infected by intracerebral inoculation of human dengue viruses and until the more recent introduction of *in vitro* cell cultures this was the preferred method for primary virus isolation. However, the full "adaptation" of dengue viruses to the mouse is not necessarily an easy task. KIMURA and HOTTA (1944) established three mouse-adapted strains of virus from the dengue epidemics in Japan in 1943 and 1944 (for detailed summary see HOTTA, 1965, 1969).

Independently, SABIN and SCHLESINGER (1945) succeeded in adapting the Hawaiian strain recovered during a 1944 dengue epidemic. These strains have been maintained until the present time as dengue-1 prototype strains.

Strains representing type 2 were also isolated during World War II from an epidemic in New Guinea (SABIN and SCHLESINGER, 1945; SABIN, 1952a), but these were successfully propagated in mice only after it was recognized that the use of newborn mice facilitated the process (MEIKLEJOHN *et al.*, 1952a; SCHLESINGER and FRANKEL, 1952a). This was followed by the adaptation of dengue-3 and -4 prototype strains isolated during epidemics of hemorrhagic fever in the Philippine Islands (HAMMON *et al.*, 1960a, b; 1964a) and by the subsequent routine isolation, by passage in newborn mice, of many strains in different parts of the world. Some strains of virus defy attempts at primary isolation in mice. For example, it was the experience of several laboratories during the dengue epidemic in the Caribbean Islands that this method failed where primary isolation in monkey kidney cell cultures succeeded (RUSSELL *et al.*, 1966b; GRIFFITHS *et al.*, 1968). SPENCE *et al.* (1969) were unable to maintain viral activity in suckling mice after intracerebral inoculation of 145 acute phase human serum specimens, nor did inoculated mice subsequently challenged with dengue-2 virus show resistance. These authors used up to 12 intracerebral blind passages and more than 600 groups of mice. Their single positive result *in mice* resulted from transfer to 1—2 day old mice of a type 3 strain first propagated in African green monkey kidney cell cultures, but it required 11 serial intracerebral passages before paralytic disease occurred. These difficulties are quite reminiscent of those encountered by SABIN and SCHLESINGER (1945) in their initial work on type 1 virus. Except as noted above, the "challenge resistance" test, using superinfection with a mouse-adapted strain especially in early passages where mice inoculated with primary or blind passage material show no signs of illness, can be an extremely useful indicator of the continued presence and activity of the suspect interfering virus (cf. HAMMON *et al.*, 1957).

Several factors influence the ease of adaptation to mice: (1) Suckling mice are more susceptible to dengue viruses than adults (MEIKLEJOHN *et al.*, 1952a; SCHLESINGER and FRANKEL, 1952a). Possible mechanisms involved in the differential responses of mice of varying age will be discussed in Section IX on Variation. (2) Different strains of mice have different degrees of susceptibility to dengue viruses. For instance, one albino strain (PRI) was reportedly more resistant to dengue virus than were Swiss mice, and the latter were less susceptible to the same virus than was the "dba" strain (SABIN and SCHLESINGER, 1945).

SABIN (1952b, c, 1954) subjected PRI and Swiss albino mice to detailed genetic analysis and found that resistance of PRI mice (= depression of viral multiplication) was inherited as a dominant autosomal trait in accord with Mendelian laws. Interestingly enough, resistance was exhibited by these mice not only to dengue but also to other group B, *but not group A*, arboviruses. This genetically controlled resistance is carried over from the intact animals to primary cell cultures derived from them (see Table 18).

Table 18. *Growth of dengue-2 virus in Swiss and PRI mouse brain fragment cultures (roller tubes)*

Exp.	Time after infection (days)	No. of fluid changes[a]	Log LD$_{50}$[b] in medium		
			Control (no tissue)	Swiss	PRI
I	0	0	3.8	n.t.[d]	n.t.
	2	0	<0.3[c]	1.6	<0.3
	5	1	n.t.	3.5	<0.3
	8	2	n.t.	3.0	<0.7[e]
II	0	0	n.t.	3.0	3.0
	4	0	n.t.	1.7	1.5
	7	1	n.t.	3.0	<0.7[e]

Fragments of suckling brain tissue were planted in glass tubes with medium consisting of 70% Earle's salt solution, 10% chick embryo extract, 20% heat-inactivated horse serum. After attachment of fragments, the tubes were placed in the roller drum. Outgrowth was observed and cultures were infected 1 week after start. Virus was dengue-2 New Guinea "B", 55th suckling mouse brain passage. 0.1 ml of a 10^{-3} dilution of stock virus was added to 0.9 ml of medium.

[a] At each fluid change 0.9 ml was replaced, resulting in 10-fold dilution.
[b] Titrations in weanling Swiss mice.
[c] No death among 5 mice inoculated with 10^{-1} medium.
[d] Not tested.
[e] 1 of 5 mice inoculated with 10^{-1} medium died.

(Unpublished results of J. W. WINTER and R. W. SCHLESINGER, 1955.)

SABIN and SCHLESINGER (1945) thought that "adaptation" to the mouse might be facilitated by the initial inoculation of virus concentrated by ultracentrifugation and then diluted. Although their early results did not bear out the expectation that this procedure might eliminate an "inhibitor" present in whole serum, the use of relatively dilute inocula—both of the initiating human serum and of subsequent mouse brain passage materials—was subsequently shown to offer advantages. But what seems to be involved in the main is the genetic heterogeneity of viral populations, resulting in "autointerference" when large doses of virus are inoculated (see Section IX on Variation).

Prior to complete "adaptation" of dengue viruses to mice, inoculated animals may show various signs of illness, ranging from ill-defined weakness of extremities or generalized debility and tremor to frank paralysis. After a number of passages, all mice suffer paralysis of the extremities and, ultimately, death (SABIN and SCHLESINGER, 1945; further details presented in SABIN, 1952a). With increasing "adaptation", the time of onset of disease and of death becomes stabilized.

Major gross pathological changes seen in the infected mice are congestion, especially in the brain and lungs. Small petechiae are often noted on the meninges or on the surface of the lungs. Hemorrhagic diathesis, of varying degrees, is generally recognized in many organs. Histologically, there are alterations which apparently correspond to the clinical signs: (1) in brain and spinal cord, cell infiltration, especially perivascular cuffing, and glial proliferation are seen, and the nerve cells exhibit degeneration; (2) in the lungs, congestion of the capillary vessels, extravasation of erythrocytes into the alveolar lumens are noted, and there are pictures characteristic of interstitial pneumonitis; (3) in the spleen and lymph nodes, activation of follicles and hyperplasia of lymphoid and reticuloendothelial cells are observed that are considered to be a reaction to generalized infection; (4) in many organs, generally, the walls of arterioles and venules are affected, revealing swelling and proliferation of vascular endothelial cells.

Typical examples of these histopathologic alterations may be found in articles by CRAIGHEAD et al. (1966) and by HOTTA (1969). A study in which the histopathologic changes at various infection stages were examined (HOTTA, 1951) indicated that, among the above-mentioned findings, the vascular changes and those in the interstitial tissues of the lungs preceded the changes in the brain and spinal cord.

Immunofluorescent tests reveal specific dengue antigens localized in the cytoplasm of nerve cells and glial cells in the brains of infected mice (BHAMARAPRAVATI et al., 1964; ATCHISON et al., 1966). Ultrastructural studies of neurons in dengue-2 infected suckling mouse brain show cytopathic effects and viral morphogenesis essentially comparable to those seen in in vitro cell cultures (SRIURAIRATNA et al., 1973).

Associated leukocytic reactions were noted in the peripheral blood of infected mice (HOTTA and SHIOMI, 1952). Compared with reactions in control mice injected intracerebrally with normal mouse brain homogenates, dengue-infected mice showed: (1) a relative tendency toward neutrophilia and lymphopenia, (2) decrease or disappearance of eosinophils, (3) marked increase of monocytes, and (4) decrease of the average nuclear number, i.e., shift to the left, of neutrophils.

C. Other Mammals

While many reports in the literature dealing with primary inoculation of human dengue virus into various laboratory animals described only negative or questionable results (cf. SIMMONS *et al.*, 1931), the following exceptions are noted:

BLANC *et al.* (1928) stated that an inapparent infection with viremia was produced in guinea pigs by injection of human dengue virus; volunteers inoculated with the blood from the infected animals were said to have developed dengue symptoms.

Several groups of investigators claimed to have noted turbidity of the lens of rabbits after injection of human dengue virus into the anterior chamber of the eye (ISHII *et al.*, 1943; KAWACHI, 1943; KUWAJIMA *et al.*, 1943; TODA *et al.*, 1943).

According to HIROKI *et al.* (1944), a species of ground squirrel (*Citellus mongolicus ramosus* Thomas) was infected with dengue virus by intracerebral or intranasal inoculation, exhibiting congestion and hemorrhage in the lungs; the virus was transmitted serially in the animals by intranasal instillation using infected lung or brain homogenates. The virus from the 5th and 14th squirrel passages was reported to have induced dengue syndromes in human volunteers. The same authors also mentioned that the virus could be transmitted to squirrels of another species *(Cricetulus griseus)* which became a carrier of the virus for a period of time without showing recognizable signs of illness.

TSURUMI and SHIN (1943) claimed that albino rats were infected with human dengue virus by intraperitoneal injection or by intranasal instillation, showing congestion and hemorrhage of the lungs.

Acceptance of these claims as evidence for specific dengue viral activity would be hazardous. During World War II, SABIN and SCHLESINGER (summarized in SABIN, 1952a) carried out numerous attempts to demonstrate evidence for maintenance of virus in hamsters, newborn and adult guinea pigs, cotton rats, and rabbits after inoculation of 5 different *bona fide* strains. None was obtained. On the other hand, it has been reported that 2 to 5-day old hamsters (MEIKLEJOHN *et al.*, 1952b) and a species of cave bat *(Myotus lucifugus)* (REAGAN and BRUECK-NER, 1952b) can be infected intracerebrally with mouse-passaged strains of dengue-1 and -2 viruses.

D. Chick Embryos

The cultivation of dengue virus in fertilized chicken eggs was claimed by SHORTT *et al.* (1936) who inoculated patient's serum onto the chorio-allantoic membrane and found macroscopic lesions such as thickening and/or pock formation; histologically, cellular proliferation on the mesodermal layer and presence of inclusion-like bodies in the cytoplasm of the affected cells were noted. During World War II, KONO (1942) in Burma, KIMURA *et al.* (1942, 1944) and KAWAMURA *et al.* (1943a, b) in the Japanese Main Islands, as well as KOBAYASHI *et al.* (1943) in Formosa (Taiwan), independently reported results essentially similar to those by SHORTT *et al.* and also claimed to have induced typical dengue syndromes by injecting healthy volunteers with emulsions of the virus-infected membranes.

Studies by other investigators, however, were not compatible with the above findings. For example, TANIGUCHI *et al.* (1943, 1951) and MISAO *et al.* (1943)

considered the chorio-allantoic lesions to be nonspecific, being produced similarly in control eggs inoculated with nonpathogenic materials such as sterile saline. Even the latter groups reported, however, that typical dengue syndromes could be induced by injecting healthy volunteers with homogenates of dengue-inoculated membranes harboring no macroscopic alterations. It seems possible, therefore, that some strains of human dengue virus may be able to persist for certain periods of time or even multiply in the chorioallantoic membrane. In the light of later findings, however, this seems unlikely.

SABIN and SCHLESINGER (unpublished, summarized in SCHLESINGER, 1950), working with five strains of dengue-1 and -2 viruses in the form of infectious human sera, made numerous attempts to demonstrate maintenance or growth of virus in embryonated eggs of different ages inoculated by various routes and incubated for varying periods at different temperatures. Materials harvested after two or more passages were inoculated into human volunteers, and in no case was virus detectable by this method.

The likelihood that these latter observations, rather than the earlier ones referred to above, have general validity is strengthened by the circumstances which finally led to the successful propagation of dengue-1 virus in embryonated eggs (SCHLESINGER, 1950, 1951). After numerous attempts to maintain virus derived from relatively low mouse passage levels in chick embryos had failed, a new series was initiated with virus that had undergone 101 intracerebral transfers in mice. Optimal results were obtained by inoculating 5-day old embryos via "peri-embryonic stab" (presumably equivalent to yolk or amniotic sac), incubating the eggs at 35° C, and harvesting whole embryos after 7 days. The titer of virus in the embryo was equivalent to that attained in the brain of weanling mice, and it multiplied to that level (about $10^{6.5}$ LD_{50}/gm) through over 90 serial passages. Once well established in eggs, incubation at 39° C gave titers equivalent to those at 35° C. Of greatest interest were the following observations: (1) by far the highest titer of virus was found in the central nervous system of chick embryos; (2) no histopathological lesions were found in the brain or spinal cord; (3) infection failed to interfere with growth and development of the embryos or with their hatchability; (4) virus could be recovered from the brains and spinal cords of chicks for at least 9—10 days after hatching (SCHLESINGER, 1951); (5) after 38 passages in chick embryos, the virus retained the attenuated character of its mouse-adapted progenitor in that two nephrotic children inoculated with it as a possible therapeutic measure suffered no or mild (low-grade fever for 2 days and rash) ill effects but produced neutralizing antibody (SCHLESINGER, 1950).

It should be mentioned that NAKAGAWA and SHINGU (1958) reported growth of mouse-adapted dengue-1 virus (Hawaii) in one-day old chick embryos some of which died about 6 days after inoculation.

E. Mosquitoes

A requirement for dengue virus replication in *Aedes aegypti* prior to its transmissibility to man was inferred from the extrinsic incubation period which lasts 8—14 days (SILER et al., 1926). SIMMONS et al. (1931) showed that *Aedes aegypti* transmitted dengue for up to 70 days after a bloodmeal, and BLANC and CAMINO-

PETROS (1930) had shown that they remained infective for 174 days. Mosquitoes are exceedingly susceptible to minute doses of dengue viruses by intrathoracic inoculation (COLEMAN and McLEAN, 1973; McLEAN et al., 1974; ROSEN and GUBLER. 1974). Under these conditions, virus replication can be demonstrated in terms of infectivity of whole ground-up mosquitoes throughout the extrinsic incubation period; its rate at temperatures below 27° C is significantly decreased (COLEMAN and McLEAN, 1973). The titers to which either human or mouse- and tissue culture-adapted virus of all 4 serotypes multiplies is at least equivalent to or greater than the titer in suckling mouse brain or in LLC-MK2 cell cultures (ROSEN and GUBLER, 1974; GUBLER and ROSEN, 1976). No evidence for pathological findings in mosquitoes has been reported.

IX. Viral Variation, Genetics

A particularly intriguing aspect of the dengue viruses is the extraordinary extent to which they acquire a predilection for growth in the central nervous system (CNS) after "adaptation" to the mouse. Studies to be summarized in this section show that the acquisition of this trait is a process probably involving more than one mutational and selective step. It manifests itself, first, in the ability of the virus to grow in, and produce disease referable to, the CNS of newborn mice; second, in the gradual emergence of a similar capacity for growth and pathological effects in adult mice. Coincident with the first step is the diminution of pathogenicity for man (attenuation), while the stabilization of neurovirulence for the mouse in the second phase seems to be associated with the ability of the virus to grow in the CNS of other hosts, viz., the monkey and the chick embryo. That the transition from the first to the second phase involves a modification in the viral genome is suggested by previously unpublished results which will be presented below. It is implicit in this statement that these studies were concerned with the behavior of populations of heterogeneous viral particles, not of cloned stocks. It should be noted at the outset that this approach suffers from the lack of clearly defined multiple genetic markers and test systems and that the results merely illustrate the need for systematic genetic studies on dengue viruses.

A. The Evolution of Neurovirulence

A systematic study of the variation of dengue-2 virus (New Guinea B strain) resulting from mouse-to-mouse passages was carried out by SCHLESINGER and FRANKEL (1952a, b; unpublished observations). The results can be summarized as follows:

(1) After an initial series of 4 intracerebral passages in weanling dba mice, some of which showed weakness or paralysis of extremities, fourth passage brain tissue was used, after 6 years of storage in the lyophilized state, to initiate a continued series of serial transfers in 1 to 7 day old-Swiss mice. From the second (total: sixth) passage onward, the lethal titer of the virus ranged between $10^{8.5}$ and 10^{10} LD_{50} per gm of suckling mouse (sm) brain tissue. Titrations showed no evidence of "autointerference" but gave predictable, sharp regressions of mortality rates.

(2) In contrast, the "dose response" of 3—4 week old weanling mice (weight 8—10 gm) was highly unpredictable up to the 24th sm passage. The contrasting behavior of the virus in mice of the two age ranges is illustrated by the summary in Fig. 27. It should be stressed that this graph gives *morbidity* rather than mortality ratios because many of the weanling mice at this intermediate stage of "adaptation" became paralyzed but survived (see Table 19). It was, however, a consistent finding that the highest incidence of illness or death occurred in groups of weanling mice inoculated with virus at relatively high dilutions (see also BANERJEE, 1969a).

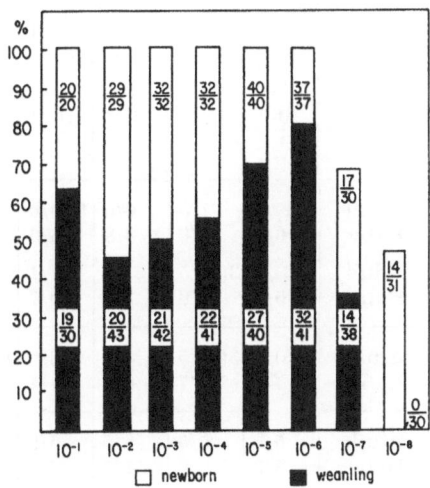

Fig. 27. Dengue-2 virus, New Guinea B strain: Cumulative incidence of CNS signs among suckling (□—□) and weanling (■—■) mice inoculated intracerebrally with indicated dilutions of virus suspensions derived from the 6th to 21st suckling mouse passages. Fractions indicate mice with paralysis in numerator, total number observed in denominator. Modified from SCHLESINGER and FRANKEL, 1952a

Table 19. *Titration in adult mice of dengue-2 virus, suckling mouse brain passage 8*

Dilution of virus inoc.	Morbidity[a]	Mortality
10^{-1}	3/8	3/8
10^{-2}	2/8	2/8
10^{-3}	3/8	1/8
10^{-4}	1/7	0/7
10^{-5}	3/8	2/8
10^{-6}	5/8	3/8
10^{-7}	1/8	0/8
10^{-8}	0/7	0/7

[a] Number of mice showing paralysis or other signs of CNS involvement/No. observed. Unpublished experiment by FRANKEL and SCHLESINGER (1952).

(3) From the 25th sm passage onward, the virus was equally pathogenic and lethal for suckling and weanling mice. However, the titer to which the virus multiplied in brains of the older mice was 10- to 100-fold lower than in those of suckling mice.

(4) "Adaptation" to weanling mice was not hastened by serial intracerebral passage in animals of that age even though multiplication of the sm-pathogenic virus was clearly demonstrable. This is illustrated in Table 20.

Table 20. *Serial passages in adult mice: comparative infectivity titrations of infected adult mouse brains in adult and in baby mice*

Adult passage series	No. of passages in adult mice	Total No. of passages in mice	Age of mice used for titration	Mortality (and Morbidity)[a] rates after inoculation of indicated dilutions							Log LD$_{50}$
				10^{-1}	10^{-2}	10^{-3}	10^{-4}	10^{-5}	10^{-6}	10^{-7}	
A	Ad. 3	9	Adult	0(1)/4	1/5	0/5	1(2)/5	2/5	—	—	b
			Baby	6/6	6/6	8/8	5/5	6/6	—	—	>5.5
	Ad. 6	12	Adult	1(3)/3	3(4)/5	0(3)/5	1/4	0(1)/5	0/5	0/5	b
			Baby	5/5	5/6	3/7	0/7	0/3	0/2	0/9	2.8
B	Ad. 6	26	Adult	4(5)/5	3(5)/5	5/5	2/5	1(2)/5	0/5	0/5	b
			Baby	4/4	7/7	6/6	4/4	2/6	0/7	0/5	4.8
C	Ad. 6	27	Adult	5/5	5/5	5/5	5/5	3/3	1/5	—	5.6
			Baby	3/3	6/6	7/7	6/6	7/7	3/6	—	6.0

[a] Figures in parentheses indicate, in addition to those mice which died, those which were sacrificed when showing CNS signs or which survived for 21 days although showing typical CNS signs for many days.

b LD$_{50}$ not calculated because of irregular results.

From SCHLESINGER and FRANKEL (1952a). With permission of the American Journal of Tropical Medicine and Hygiene.

(5) The same patterns of age-dependence were demonstrable with RNA extracted with phenol from mouse brains infected with "high" or "low" passage dengue-2 virus, respectively (SCHULZE, 1962). Here, the former yielded clean titration end points in test animals of either age (about 10^{-5} that of the virus source). In contrast, titrations of virus or RNA from a "low" passage (sm 10) gave the results shown in Fig. 28. These results suggested that the change in the viral properties responsible for the increased virulence for adult mice resided in the viral genome.

(6) The findings summarized thus far led to the working hypothesis that viral populations up to the passage level where virulence for adult mice finally became fixed, were mixtures of two classes of particles, *i.e.*, those which were pathogenic for suckling mice only and those which were pathogenic for mice of either age (SCHLESINGER and FRANKEL, 1952a). It was postulated that the titration patterns in adult mice shown in Figs. 27 and 28 could be explained by assuming that high proportions of the nonpathogenic component could effectively protect mice by

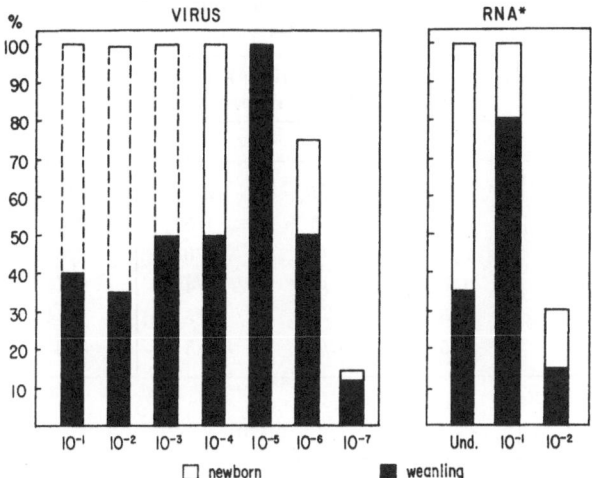

Fig. 28. Dengue-2 virus, New Guinea B strain: Mortality rates in suckling (□—□) and weanling (■—■) mice inoculated intracerebrally with indicated dilutions of virus derived from suckling mouse brain passage 10 or of RNA isolated therefrom by three sequential cold phenol extractions. (Broken lines in "newborn" columns at 10^{-1} to 10^{-3} indicate that these dilutions were not included in this experiment, but see Fig. 27)

* No infectivity recovered after treatment with ribonuclease, 5 μg/ml, for 20 minutes at room temp. Similar treatment had no effect on infectivity of whole virus. "Undiluted RNA" was equivalent v/v to 20% brain extract.
Modified from SCHULZE (1962)

interfering with the virulent component and that this effect was reduced by dilution of the inoculum.

(7) This hypothesis was tested by reconstruction experiments which showed clearly that low passage virus, in mixtures with high passage virus, could interfere with the lethal effects of the latter (SCHLESINGER and FRANKEL, 1952b). Interference was enhanced by allowing increasing time intervals between the interfering and the challenge virus (Table 21). Similar basic observations were recorded by COLE and WISSEMAN (1969a) who related the protective activity to (a) differential rates of multiplication of the two viral test populations, (b) rate of interferon induction, (c) rate of antibody response.

(8) From the point of view of possible genetic implications of these early findings, the following two types of observations are of interest:

(a) As shown in Table 22, "low passage" viral RNA simulated the interfering effect of the virus from which it was derived (SCHLESINGER and SCHULZE, unpublished data);

(b) A remarkable "rescue" of the virulence marker was encountered in checkerboard titrations in which different amounts of interfering low passage virus were mixed with varying amounts of high passage challenge virus. As shown in Table 23, a mortality rate far in excess of the additive rate induced by the two component virus populations alone occurred among those mice inoculated with mixtures containing various doses of *low* passage virus with a sublethal dose of high passage

Table 21. *Interference by "low passage" with "high passage" dengue-2 virus in adult mice : variation in time interval*[a]

Passage s.m. 38, dilution inoculated	Interval (days) between "low" and "high" passage inoculum				s.m. 38 control
	0	1	3	5	
10^{-3}	5/5	3/4	2/5	0/4	—
10^{-4}	5/5	4/5	1/5	0/4	—
10^{-5}	3/5	2/5	1/5	2/5	20/20
10^{-6}	1/5	1/4	0/4	0/4	20/20
10^{-7}	1/5	1/5	1/5	1/4	19/20
10^{-8}	1/5	0/4	0/5	0/5	4/19
No s.m. 38, s.m. 8 control	2/20				

[a] "Low passage" virus: 10^{-3} suckling mice brain from passage 8.
   "High passage" virus: suckling mice brain passage 38.
Data reported in SCHLESINGER and FRANKEL (1952b).

Table 22. *Intracerebral interference by dengue-2 "low passage RNA" with "high passage" virus — 4 day interval*[a]

s.m. passage 10 RNA dilution	s.m. passage 58 virus						s.m. 10 RNA only
	10^{-4}	10^{-5}	10^{-6}	10^{-7}	10^{-8}	10^{-9}	
Undil.[b]	5/5	5/5	1/5	0/5	2/5	1/5	4/7
10^{-1}	4/5	2/2	4/4	5/5	3/5	4/5	4/5
10^{-2}	5/5	4/4	4/4	4/5	1/5	1/5	0/4
None, s.m. passage 58 only	6/6	6/6	5/5	3/5	0/5	0/5	—

[a] RNA was extracted from suckling mouse (s.m.) brain representing passage 10 by 3 cold phenol extractions (SCHULZE, 1962). Adult mice inoculated with RNA at dilutions indicated were challenged 4 days later with s.m. passage 68 stock virus.
[b] "Undil. RNA" is equivalent v/v to 20% mouse brain extract.
SCHULZE and SCHLESINGER, unpublished data (1962).

virus (SCHLESINGER and FRANKEL, 1952, unpublished experiments). Again, similar experiments carried out with low passage virus and high passage RNA suggested a similar trend (SCHLESINGER and SCHULZE, 1961, unpublished experiments).

These results would be most readily explicable by the assumption that, in varying dosage ranges, there may occur interference in one or the other direction or, alternatively, complementation or recombination. Clarification of the latter alternatives will have to await the development of viral clones with mutant markers more easily defined and scored than are different levels of neurovirulence, *e.g.*, temperature sensitivity.

BANERJEE (1969) and COLE and WISSEMAN (1969b) have presented evidence connecting high neurovirulence to capacity of dengue virus to grow at high tem-

Table 23. *Intracerebral inoculation of mixtures of "high passage" and "low passage" type 2 dengue virus in weanling mice*[a]

Ratio "high"/"low"[b]	Dilution of "high passage" virus in mixture							"Low passage" only —
	10^{-3}	10^{-4}	10^{-5}	10^{-6}	10^{-7}	10^{-8}	10^{-9}	All dilutions
10^{-2}	7/13[c]	5/6	10/14	4/6	7/13	4/6	4/5	
10^{-3}	—	4/14	2/6	7/13	3/5	7/14	4/5	41/128 (32%)
10^{-4}	—	—	1/12	2/6	3/14	3/5	11/12	
10^{-5}	—	—	—	0/5	1/6	0/6	4/5	
Total dead	7/13	9/20	13/32	13/30	14/38	14/31	23/27	— —
% dead	53	45	40	43	37	45	85	— —
"High passage" only	28/28	28/28	28/28	26/26	11/27	3/28	0/26	— —
% dead	100	100	100	100	41	10	0	— —

[a] Combined data from two separate experiments. Viruses used were in the form of suckling mouse (s. m.) brain suspensions. "Low passage" virus: s. m. passage 8 (Exp. I) and 9 (Exp. II). "High passage" virus: s. m. passage 37 (Exp. I) and 51 (Exp. II).

[b] Ratio "high"/"low" reflects the ten-fold dilutions of the two respective virus preparations mixed prior to inoculation. The actual dilution of the "low" passage virus in each mixture can be calculated from the ratio and the dilution of "high" passage virus. Thus, at "high" passage dilution 10^{-9} the "low" passage virus was added at 10^{-7} (ratio 10^{-2}), 10^{-6} (ratio 10^{-3}), etc. Corresponding mortality rates for the "low" passage virus used in the 10^{-9} column were:

$$\text{LP } 10^{-7} \quad 5/12 = 42\%$$
$$\text{LP } 10^{-6} \quad 5/11 = 45\%$$
$$\text{LP } 10^{-5} \quad 9/28 = 32\%$$
$$\text{LP } 10^{-4} \quad 6/12 = 50\%$$
$$\text{Total} \quad 25/63 = 40\%$$

[c] Number of mice dead/number inoculated.

Based on unpublished observations by R. W. Schlesinger, J. W. Frankel, and J. W. Winter (1951—53).

perature. Dengue and the other group B togaviruses are ripe for intensive genetic analysis through use of ts mutants, but only limited systematic work along these lines has so far been reported (Tarr and Lubiniecki, 1975, 1976).

The conclusion that stabilization of neurovirulence is an expression of a genetic change in the virus is supported by the fact, already cited, that its manifestation in the adult mouse is paralleled by very striking increases in neurotropism in the monkey (Sabin, 1955), chick embryo (Schlesinger, 1951) and, apparently, in the hamster (Meiklejohn et al., 1952b). This type of organ-specific adaptation, crossing, as it does, the barrier between diverse species, is a subject of unique interest in relation to the evolution of changing patterns in viral pathogenicity. The association of these modifications with altered pathogenicity for the natural host of dengue viruses—man—underlines this conclusion.

B. Attenuation of Human Pathogenicity

Whenever mouse-adapted strains of dengue-1 or -2 viruses have been inoculated into human volunteers, it has been confirmed that they had lost the capacity of producing typical dengue fever but retained their immunizing capacity (SABIN and SCHLESINGER, 1945; HOTTA, 1952; SABIN, 1955; SCHLESINGER et al., 1956). In the case of the Hawaiian strain (type 1), SABIN and SCHLESINGER (1945) reported that virus from the first 6 mouse passages induced fairly severe types of experimental infection, while later passage levels produced either no or very mild systemic reactions (fever for 1—2 days with or without headache and malaise) starting 8—10 days after inoculation. The only constant finding was an extensive maculo-papular rash, often followed by petechiae on feet and ankles. This modified infection was followed by the development of solid immunity to challenge with homologous unmodified (human) virus. *Aedes aegypti* feeding on volunteers during the acute phase of the modified reaction became infected with some difficulty and then transmitted the virus in its attenuated form to other volunteers. Further work toward the development of a dengue-1 vaccine from this attenuated strain has been reported by WISSEMAN et al. (1963) [see Section XI (Immunization)].

Essentially similar findings were obtained by KIMURA and HOTTA with the Mochizuki strain of dengue-1 which they had adapted to mice in 1943—1944 (cf. HOTTA, 1952, 1965, 1969). However, full attenuation of this strain required over 30 serial passages in mice.

As already mentioned, the attenuated character of the Hawaiian strain of dengue-1 virus was retained after 38 passages in chick embryos initiated with 101st mouse passage virus (SCHLESINGER, 1950).

Type 2 virus (New Guinea C strain), subjected to 18 mouse passages (MEIKLE-JOHN et al., 1952a), was tested in human volunteers by SABIN (1955) who observed no clinical manifestations other than rash and the formation of neutralizing antibody. Similarly, SCHLESINGER et al. (1956) carried out tests in human volunteers with the New Guinea B strain that had undergone 40 to 46 passages in mice (SCHLESINGER and FRANKEL, 1952a). With exception of very minor brief temperature elevations in about one-half of the patients, rashes, and some leukopenia, there were no clinical reactions but effective antibody production in 10 of the 11 men. Virus could be recovered from only one of the 11 volunteers and it proved to be of the modified kind (SCHLESINGER et al., 1956).

Additional aspects of attenuated dengue viruses, particularly those relating to immunological responses of man and animals to sequential infection with different flaviviruses, will be discussed in Section XI.

X. Essential Clinical Features

A. General Considerations

Two distinct clinical entities are associated with dengue virus infections of man. These are (A) "classical" or *primary* dengue fever, (B) dengue hemorrhagic fever (DHF) (with or without shock) or *secondary* dengue. Usage of the terms "primary" and "secondary" denotes that the clinical outcome of an infection may be critically influenced by the patient's previous experience with dengue virus. A large body of epidemiological evidence, reinforced by laboratory data, does indeed suggest that DHF and the dengue shock syndrome (DSS) are characteristic complications of secondary exposure under specialized conditions affecting mainly children in heavily endemic regions. Nevertheless, the occasional association of similarly severe syndromes in individuals with *primary* dengue fever has been reported as well. These reports are not, *a priori*, incompatible with a unified concept of pathogenetic mechanisms based on immunological phenomena. However, the immune state of a *population at risk* and the viral-ecological environment in which it finds itself seem to have a great deal to do with the disease patterns one can expect. Therefore clinical features will be discussed in a single context with basic virological and immunological facts as well as with epidemiological variables. In light of the subjects covered in the preceding chapters or of generally accepted principles, the following are some of the obvious factors that come to mind as possibly playing a role:

(a) *The virus:* The four types of dengue virus differ from one another by virtue of type-specific antigenic determinants; they share some (dengue) subgroup-specific determinant and, in addition, possess the group-specific antigen(s) carried by all group B togaviruses. Within certain types, the evolution of antigenically modified subtypes has been documented (see Section VI. E). Is antigenic structure related to "virulence" for man? Are there other measurable properties (*e.g.*, "adaptability" to experimental host systems, thermostability) associated with one or another kind of pathogenic propensity?

(b) *The immune state:* How does previous experience with one dengue type modify the response to infection with the same or heterologous types? Can similar modification result from past exposure to *any* group B togavirus? Can the intervention of an evolving immune response, even in primary dengue, express itself in the form of immunopathological complications?

(c) *The population at risk:* Dengue fever occurs in *epidemic* form when the virus is introduced into an environment in which it can establish itself by virtue of the presence of *Aedes* vectors and a susceptible human population. In such a situation, one sees explosive outbreaks of primary disease, usually initiated by a single antigenic type. Such an episode can either wane as quickly as it spread, or it can lead to the *endemic* establishment of the virus. What happens when the same population is exposed to epidemic introduction of homotypic or heterotypic virus or when monotypic endemicity is amplified by the endemic establishment of other virus types? Does the passage of time affect the status and the response of the population? Are there definable factors other than the immune state—age, sex, race, nutrition, etc.—which predispose to one or the other kind of clinical response (classical dengue vs. DHF or DSS)?

(d) *The vector:* As has been discussed (cf. Table 2), various members of the genus *Aedes* (Stegomyia) are capable of transmitting dengue virus. The chief vector of *urban* dengue is *Aedes aegypti*, a domestic species, that of *sylvan* dengue probably *Aedes albopictus*, an inhabitant of rain forests. Do these different mosquito species impose on the virus distinct selective pressures that imprint different pathogenic properties? Are these properties further influenced by the rapidity of transmission, *i.e.*, by the density of vector and susceptible human populations? The persistence of virus in infected mosquitoes during their adult lifespan has

been discussed in previous chapters. There is evidence from work on other togaviruses for the selective emergence of ts and other mutant characters in chronically
infected mosquito cell cultures (cf. SHENK et al., 1974; STOLLAR et al., 1974); the
occurrence of similar phenomena in nature could have a profound effect on patterns
of pathogenicity (SCHLESINGER, 1975). These patterns would be influenced further
by the ambient temperature, by the lifespan of infected female mosquitoes, by
breeding and hibernating habits, etc.

(e) *Intermediate hosts:* Observations in nature as well as under laboratory conditions indicate that certain species of monkeys can serve as alternate hosts for
dengue viruses (see Section VIII. A.). Under natural conditions, a major role
could be assigned to simian hosts only in rain forests, where presumably *A. albopictus* is the chief vector. The question therefore arises whether such a sylvan
alternative to the urban *A. aegypti*—man—*A. aegypti*—man ... cycle could
contribute to modifications of pathogenic properties.

It should be emphasized that, with a few exceptions, hard evidence bearing
on the possible role of these variables is lacking. But an awareness of such general
considerations may aid in the presentation and understanding of clinical data
and obviates the need to provide an encyclopedic catalogue of *all* available clinical
and epidemiological permutations that have been recorded.

B. Primary "Classical Dengue Fever"

1. Clinical Course and Clinical Laboratory Findings

The following is a brief synthesis of textbook descriptions of "typical" dengue
fever seen in natural cases or experimentally infected young adult Caucasian male
volunteers (SABIN 1948a, 1952d, 1959; SCHLESINGER, 1958; HAMMON, 1963;
HOTTA, 1969).

The incubation period averages 5—8 days from the time of bite by one or more
infected mosquitoes. The onset of illness may be preceded for a few hours by
various undifferentiated prodromata such as headache, backache, stiffness, general
malaise and flushed or mottled facial skin. The onset of more typical symptoms
is sudden, with a sharp rise in temperature associated with chilliness and severe
headache; within the first 24 hours the patient develops retroorbital pain, especially
on movement of the eyes or pressure, photophobia, backache, and pain in the
muscles and joints of the extremities. Other symptoms that are commonly found
are general extreme weakness, anorexia and constipation, altered taste sensations,
colicky pains, abdominal tenderness, drawing pains in the inguinal area and testicles,
sore throat, and general depression which may cause the patient to take a dim
view of his chances of recovery. Symptoms vary in severity from mild to excruciatingly severe and usually persist for several days, sometimes with an apparent
remission and relapse halfway through the febrile period. The temperature usually
ranges between 39° and 40° C and fever lasts, on the average, 5 to 6 days. Occasionally the temperature returns to normal about the third day, only to rise again
for another 2 or 3 days ("saddleback" fever). During the first half of the febrile
period, there is no distinctive rash, but the face, neck and chest may show diffuse
flushing or mottling or fleeting pinpoint eruptions.

About the third or fourth day, a conspicuous rash appears that may be maculo-papular or scarlatiniform. It starts on the chest and trunk and spreads to the extremities and face. Itching and dermal hyperesthesia may be accompanying the rash.

During the initial phase, the temperature and pulse rate are proportionate, but the second half of the febrile period and early convalescence are characterized by relative and sometimes absolute bradycardia. There is generalized enlargement of lymphnodes, but spleen and liver are usually not enlarged.

Toward the end of the febrile period or immediately after defervescence, as the generalized rash fades, localized clusters of pinpoint hemorrhagic lesions (petechiae) may appear over the dorsum of the feet, on the legs, hands or fingers or occasionally on the mucous membranes of the oral cavity.

Convalescence may be abrupt and uneventful, but often full recovery takes longer, sometimes several weeks, accompanied by pronounced asthenia and depression.

The most significant clinical laboratory findings during the acute illness relate to the total and differential white blood cell (WBC) count. As a rule, the total WBC count is normal at onset of fever, then leukopenia develops which lasts throughout the febrile period. Even at the beginning, there is a marked depletion of circulating lymphocytes, and the neutrophile cells show a progressive shift to the left, *i.e.*, increased proportion of immature non-segmented nuclear forms, which persists into convalescence. Thrombocyte counts are usually normal as are various other components of the blood clotting mechanism, serum enzymes and other blood chemical parameters which are altered in HF or DSS (HALSTEAD *et al.*, 1970c). The cerebrospinal fluid is normal (SABIN, 1952a).

The *pathological findings* in uncomplicated primary dengue in human volunteers have been studied only in the form of skin biopsies obtained during the appearance of maculopapular and petechial eruptions (SABIN, 1952d). In neither type of lesion was it possible to discern involvement of the epithelium or inclusions. The maculopapular lesion involved endothelial swelling of small cutaneous blood vessels, perivascular edema and infiltration with mononuclear cells. The petechiae showed extravasation of blood but negligible inflammatory reaction. Extensive degenerative and hemorrhagic lesions in various internal organs have been reported in supposedly uncomplicated fatal cases during outbreaks in Australia and Greece (cited in SABIN, 1952d; see also BARNES and ROSEN, 1974). The question of whether such cases may resemble in pathogenetic mechanism the hemorrhagic and shock manifestations of secondary dengue cannot be resolved (see below).

Variations: As mentioned, the relative duration or severity of illness varies tremendously among individuals in a given epidemic as well as from one epidemic to another. Only a few arbitrarily chosen examples of this variability will be mentioned here.

The point can be illustrated by the initial human transmission tests with the dengue-1 and -2 prototype strains isolated during World War II from epidemics in Hawaii, India, and New Guinea (SABIN, 1952a). Table 24 presents a summary which shows variations in nature and severity of clinical reactions not only among the donors but also among the recipients in the first passages. On continued passage through human volunteers, either by mosquito transmission or by intracutaneous inoculation, all seven strains produced typical dengue fever with all textbook features, including a conspicuous rash in the overwhelming majority of cases. In general, however, the type 2 strains from New Guinea produced illness of shorter duration and less severity than the Hawaiian type 1 strain.

Table 24. *Initial human transmission experiments with 7 strains of dengue virus**

Place (date) of origin	Strain destination	Antigenic type	Diagnosis and clinical features in donor patient(s)	Results of Transmission	
				No. of pts.	Severity of illness (first passage only)
Hawaii (March 1944)	Hawaii	1	"Dengue"—Pool of sera collected from 6 pts. 24—48 hours after onset	6/6[a]	+ + + +[b] *with rash*
Calcutta (Sept. 1945)	India K	1	"FUO", 5—6 d., *rash*, CSF 64 mg% protein	2/2	+ + + *without rash*
	India W	1	"Dengue", 4—5 d., *no rash*, CSF normal	1/1	+ + + + *with rash*
New Guinea (April—May 1944)	New Guinea A	1	"FUO", 2 d., *no rash* (2 donors)[c]	2/2	+ + + *with rash*
	New Guinea B	2	"Dengue", >4 d., *no rash* (2 donors)[c]	2/2	+ + + *with rash*
	New Guinea C	2		2/2	+ + + *with rash*
	New Guinea D	2		2/2	+ + + *with rash*

[a] No. of volunteers responding/No. inoculated.
[b] Arbitrary scale in terms of duration, height of fever, severity of symptoms.
[c] There is no published record identifying these four strains with their individual donors.
* Based on SABIN (1952a).

Of particularly poignant interest is the recent follow-up on the seminal studies by SILER *et al.* (1926) and SIMMONS *et al.* (1931) reported by HALSTEAD (1974). In 1971—1972 he secured serum samples from four volunteers experimentally infected in 1924—1925 with the "COLLINS" strain and five in 1929—1930 with the "KELLER" strain and found HI, CF, and neutralizing activity in most of them even in absence of subsequent exposure to flaviviruses. He concluded that the "KELLER" strain had probably been type 1, the "COLLINS" type 4. Comparison of the duration and frequency of clinical signs and symptoms suggests that the type 1 virus produced the more severe illness.

During the type 3 dengue epidemic in Puerto Rico in 1963, most of the classical symptoms were present but NEFF *et al.* (1967) noted that severe incapacitation, relapses of symptoms and prolonged convalescence with depression and lack of energy were absent. The illness in Puerto Rico was similar in children under 10 years of age and in adults. What was particularly striking during the epidemic was the large number of patients with various symptoms and signs which, on clinical grounds, could have been mistaken for mild dengue fever but could not be confirmed serologically. NEFF et al. (1967) established four clinical criteria "(a) an illness of at least three days' duration characterized by (b) fever and chilliness, (c) rash and (d) incapacitation . . . for at least two days". Serological confirmation of dengue infection was obtained in the majority of patients fulfilling all four criteria but in the minority of those meeting only two or three.

The island experienced another epidemic in 1969, this time caused by dengue-2 virus (LIKOSKY et al., 1973). Symptoms were again typical but seemed to be generally milder in children under six years of age. Rashes were seen in only about 35% of serologically confirmed cases aged 6 years or older.

In general, the Caribbean experience of the past decade (cf. EHRENKRANZ et al., 1971) is instructive in that it points up the difficulty in delimiting mild and severe extremes in the clinical variability of dengue fever on clinical grounds alone. It is axiomatic that, in the face of a widespread epidemic, the populace as well as the medical and public health professionals will identify with it miscellaneous unrelated intercurrent illnesses. It is therefore vitally important that comprehensive clinical description be refined by sorting out virologically or serologically confirmed cases from the total.

Of special interest is the "non-dengue-like" character of illness in children with primary or secondary dengue infection seen as *outpatients* in Thailand in 1962—1964 (HALSTEAD et al., 1969 a; the classification as "primary" or "secondary" rests solely on the nature of the antibody response in serologically confirmed cases; see below). Of 323 febrile native outpatients studied in detail, 94 were confirmed as dengue, 26 as chikungunya, and 212 remained etiologically unidentified. Tabulations of available information on symptoms and signs make it clear that the distinction between these three groups on clinical grounds alone could not have been made, and that the most valid clinical diagnosis for all of them would have been "fever of unknown origin" or "upper respiratory infection". The same uncharacteristic mildness of dengue fever was observed in children of foreign white families residing in Thailand, at a time when the disease in their adult compatriots had the features of "classical" dengue (HALSTEAD et al., 1969 b). Again HALSTEAD (1974) reminds us that it was SIMMONS et al., (1931) who first suggested that endemicity of dengue in the Philippine Islands was based on silent infections in native children.

Another important example of variability, even under carefully controlled conditions of experimental infection, is the incidence of hemorrhagic manifestations (petechiae, epistaxis, or more serious hemorrhagic complications) in primary dengue. Thus, it was noted that petechiae were common in volunteers infected with the Hawaiian strain of type 1 virus but not in those infected with the type 2 strains from New Guinea (SABIN, 1952 a). In a well studied outbreak among U.S. Naval personnel on a Pacific Island during World War II about 20% of the patients showed petechiae (STEWART, 1944); of 31 serologically confirmed dengue cases among American soldiers in Vietnam, 4 showed such lesions (DELLER and RUSSELL, 1967). Severe hemorrhagic complications and even fatal shock have been ascribed to primary dengue-2 infection in an explosive outbreak on a Pacific Island (Niue) which appears to have had no incursion by dengue during the preceding 25 years (BARNES and ROSEN, 1974). These authors cite similar reports. less dramatic than theirs and without documentation of fatalities, to support their view that serious hemorrhagic complications may not be limited to secondary infections [cf. also EHRENKRANZ et al. (1971) for review of hemorrhagic complications in early outbreaks of dengue in Texas (1885, 1897, 1922)]. The question is whether the occasional occurrence of these, or even of petechiae, implies that pathological permeability of bloodvessels or capillaries in the course of primary dengue may have a pathogenetic basis fundamentally related to the mechanism of hemorrhagic complications in secondary infection. The subject will be discussed further below (see Section X. C. 4.).

2. Virological Findings

Primary dengue fever can be induced in man either by the bite of one or more infected mosquitoes or by the intracutaneous inoculation of virus-containing human serum (SILER et al., 1926; SIMMONS et al., 1931; SABIN, 1952a). Since uncomplicated dengue is not a fatal disease, the distribution of virus in the organism or the site(s) of virus multiplication are unknown. Serum collected from a patient at 24 hours after onset contains 10^6 human infectious doses (MID) per ml (SABIN, 1952a; ROSEN and GUBLER, 1974), and transmission of typical illness can be achieved by intracutaneous inoculation of from 10 to 10^6 MID. One MID may induce typical dengue, a mild attack followed by immunity, or no evidence of infection (SABIN, 1952a).

Viremia probably persists at some level prior to and throughout the febrile period (cf. HALSTEAD et al., 1969b), although systematic studies on this point in uncomplicated cases have been infrequent (summarized in HALSTEAD et al., 1973c).

3. Immunity

Many of the reports referred to in Section III took advantage of the long persistence of anti-dengue antibodies to identify early epidemics through serological surveys. Further support for the notion that dengue antibodies probably persist for life comes from the recent study of 9 of SILER's and SIMMONS' volunteers whose sera were tested 42 to 48 years after their only known experience with the virus (HALSTEAD, 1974).

Under controlled conditions, i.e., in experimental infections of adult volunteers (SABIN, 1952a), recovery from primary dengue fever leads to solid and lasting protection against a second infection with the same antigenic type. The response to a challenge with a heterotypic strain depends on the time interval after the first illness. SABIN found that gradually diminishing cross protection was demonstrable between 2 and 9 months after the primary attack. Initially, protection was complete, but by the end of that period, volunteers responded with a febrile illness of 2 to 3 days' duration *without rash*. Virus could be demonstrated in the blood of such individuals.

A well-documented case of two episodes of naturally acquired dengue fever, 1 year apart, caused by type 4 and 1 virus, respectively, has been reported by

CAREY et al. (1965). This concerned an American physician who had arrived in Vellore, South India, about a year before the first attack and who had been vaccinated previously against yellow fever. The two dengue viruses were isolated from his acute phase blood samples and he showed significant antibody rises (of the anamnestic type, presumably due to the earlier yellow fever vaccination, see Section XI) in convalescence from both episodes.

It was in the study of volunteer patients that the existence of at least two antigenic types of dengue virus was initially demonstrated by intracutaneous neutralization tests (SABIN and SCHLESINGER, 1945; SABIN, 1950). This test was based on the observation that intradermal inoculation of infectious human serum led to the formation, after 3—4 days, of edema and erythema at the site of inoculation, measuring 1—4 cm in diameter. This lesion as well as the ensuing systemic disease was prevented by homotypic but not heterotypic convalescent sera (see Table 9, Section VI).

HI and CF tests on convalescent sera generally show cross reactions with the four type-specific dengue antigens but the homotypic titer tends to be 2- to 4-fold higher than heterotypic reactions (SCOTT et al., 1972). It has been shown that the IgM fraction from early convalescent sera is more type-specific in HI than the whole serum or the IgG fraction (WESTAWAY, 1968; SCOTT et al., 1972; EDELMAN and PARIYANONDA, 1973).

On the contrary, in complement fixation tests, it has been shown by SCOTT and RUSSELL (1972) that dengue-2 convalescent sera (from the 1969 epidemic in Puerto Rico) gave negative or low titers, but that the IgG fraction from such sera reacted specifically and to high titers. Addition of IgM isolated from specific immune sera (but not from control sera) strongly inhibited complement fixation by both whole serum and IgG. These results presumably reflected reaction with virion-associated antigens (BRANDT et al., 1970), since FALKLER et al. (1973) found no significant number of reactions with the nonstructural SCF antigen (see Section VI. E. 4.) in primary dengue convalescents who did possess antiviral CF and HI antibodies.

Of special interest is the question of the mutual relationship not only among the 4 dengue types but also between dengue and other group B togaviruses, as it expresses itself in human beings (or experimental animals). We have already discussed the fact that recovery from infection with one dengue serotype does not impart lasting protection against the others. Extensive work has been done on the possible utilization of antigenic group relationships among all group B viruses in the development of sequential immunization programs. Since these proposals envisage the use of attenuated dengue viruses, they will be discussed in the section on Immunization.

Although not immediately germane to the subject of *human* primary dengue, attention is called to the intriguing observation by HALSTEAD et al. (1973) to the effect that leukocytes obtained from monkeys immune to one of the dengue types can be stimulated *in vitro* by exposure to any of the four serotypes to make more virus than non-immune leukocytes. Whether this is simply a reflection of enhanced lymphoblast transformation is not clear from an addendum to the paper by HALSTEAD et al. (1973 b) indicating somewhat conflicting preliminary results on the effects of phytohemagglutinin stimulation of immune and non-immune

leukocytes on dengue virus replication. More recent experiments by Sung *et al.*
(1975) involving human lymphoblastoid cell lines will be discussed below (Section
XI. A. 1.).

C. Secondary Dengue: Dengue Hemorrhagic Fever and the Shock Syndrome

1. General Remarks

The association of "hemorrhagic fever" with dengue viruses was first observed
by Hammon *et al.* (1957, 1958, 1960a. b) during an outbreak in the Philippine
Islands in 1954. Fig. 29 shows the geographic extent of this association between
1950 and 1964 (Halstead, 1966). Halstead (1965) has summarized evidence
suggesting that, far from being a "new" disease, "syndromes characterized by
severe hemorrhage or shock and death occurring with dengue epidemics have

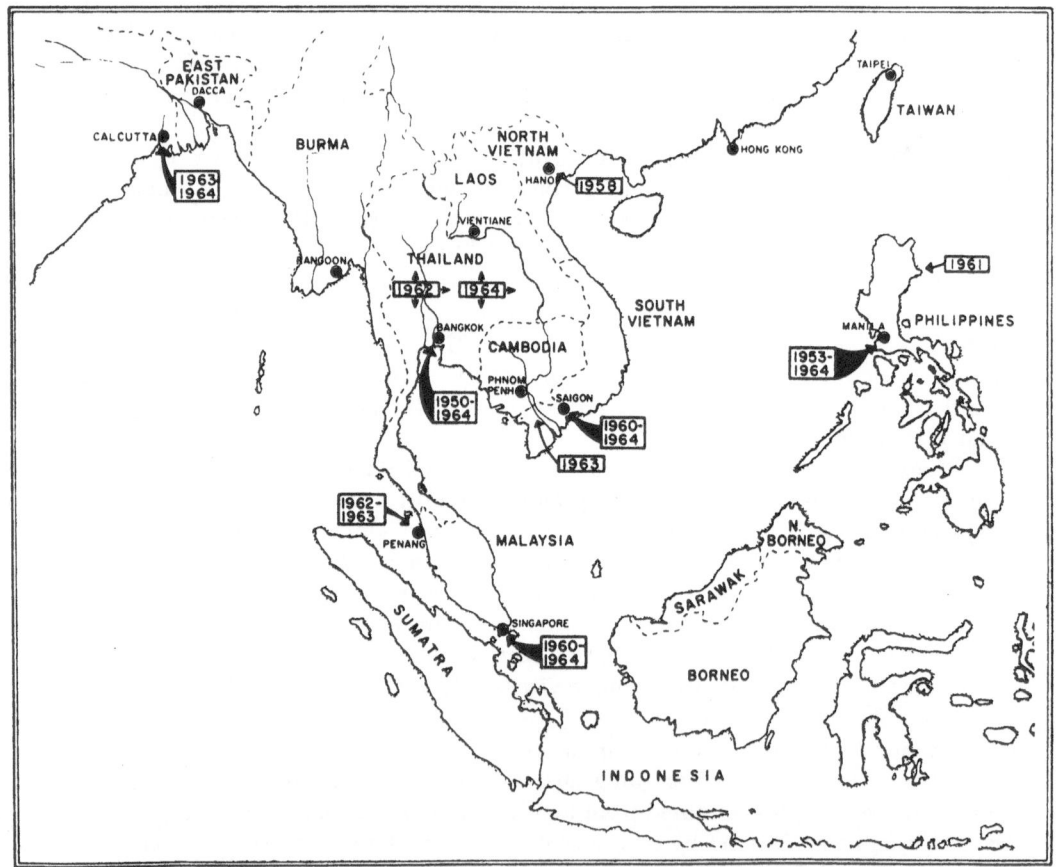

Fig. 29. Location of mosquito-borne haemorrhagic fever outbreaks in South and
Southeast Asia, 1953—64. From Halstead (1966)
With permission of the author and the Office of Publications, World Health
Organization

been described . . . in [Queensland in 1897], the Southern United States in 1922, Durban, South Africa in 1927, Greece in 1928, Formosa in 1931 . . .''. A huge volume of literature has been published since 1960 on the clinical, epidemiological and immunological features of this disease as well as on its relationship to dengue viruses and ideas about pathogenetic mechanisms. Major symposia or monographs can be found in SEATO Med. Research Monograph No. 2, Bangkok (1962), 144 pp.; Bulletin of the World Health Organization 35, No. 1, 104 pp. (1966); Jap. J. Med. Sci. Biol. 20, Suppl. 50 pp. (1967); Yale J. Biol. & Med. 42, No. 5, pp. 261—362 (1970).

Despite the historical indications cited above for previous occurrence of similar syndromes [and the more recent description by BARNES and ROSEN (1974) already referred to], there can be no question that the *pandemic* character of this complication that has prevailed in South East Asia since the early 1950's must rest on some fundamentally altered set of circumstances. Briefly, it has affected mainly *children* living in urban population centers in which *Aedes aegypti* abound and *more than one type of dengue virus* is endemic. Serological evidence indicates that affected children show a *secondary immune response* except for infants under one year of age who are believed to be immunologically conditioned by *maternal antibodies* and give a *primary* active *immune response*. In light of what is known about "classical" primary dengue and the patterns of immunity following it (see previous section), an *immunological explanation* of the phenomenon (*i. e.*, secondary infection) *must account for some special circumstances which lead to modified response rather than to one of either complete suceptibility or protection.*

2. Clinical Course and Clinical Laboratory Findings

The overall clinical course has been described as follows by HAMMON (1963): "The diseases observed in different areas have not been identical clinically; however, many similarities were noted. The common features are as follows: The onset is usually abrupt, with fever. Nausea and vomiting are common. The throat appears injected and there may be a dry cough. About the second or third day petechiae appear, usually first on the face or distal portions of the extremities but sparing the axillae and chest. The tourniquet test may be conspiciously positive before petechiae appear. Purpura and large ecchymoses as well as other manifestations of bleeding tendency are occasionally prominent. There may be severe abdominal pain and tenderness. About the third or fourth day vomiting may produce copious coffee-ground material. Melena also is not uncommon, but gross bleeding from the intestines is rare. Shock is likely to occur in severe cases about the fourth day and this critical state lasts about 12 to 24 hours. At this time the temperature falls to normal, the blood pressure is low or unmeasurable, the limbs are cool and present a purple or brownish mottled appearance. Perspiration is frequently profuse. The face and hands appear edematous. This state of shock is entirely out of proportion to the apparent loss of blood. Thrombocytopenia is noted during the period of shock, and bleeding time is prolonged. Leukocytes remain at approximately normal levels but are elevated in number more frequently than they are depressed. The leukocyte count and differential are not those observed in (primary) dengue. Although the numbers of both immature and mature polymorphonuclear cells are decreased. there is an increase in lymphocytes and sometimes in monocytes.

Differences observed between the diseases seen in the Philippines in 1956 and in Bangkok in 1958 arc: (1) Hepatomegaly was common in Bangkok, absent in Manila. (2) A deep red-purplish blush of the skin which did not blanch on pressure and pale, normal colored skin in small blotchy irregular areas was common in Manila but rare in Bangkok. This phenomenon frequently was brought on by application of a tourniquet and remained conspicuous for several days. (3) Epistaxis was very common in Manila, rare in Bangkok. Fleeting, dengue-like early and late type rashes were occasionally seen in Bangkok only, but these were missed unless searched for carefully. In Singapore in 1960 splenomegaly was a conspicuous part of the disease syndrome but this did not occur in Manila or Bangkok.

Not observed or extremely rare in all outbreaks were hematuria, heavy albuminuria, oliguria, or anuria, bleeding gums, uterine bleeding, jaundice, nuchal rigidity, paralysis, encephalitis, retroorbital pain, joint pains, swelling of joints and general lymphadenopathy (exception, Singapore).

If the patient survives the shock, recovery is very prompt and ordinarily is not followed by a period of asthenia or depression. Total duration of fever and illness is usually five to seven days.

Milder cases without bleeding tendencies or shock and of shorter duration are frequently observed. These are characterized essentially by fever only."

The authors of a report of an international collaborative study conducted in 1971 in Bangkok (WHO Report, 1973) adopted the following classification of dengue hemorrhagic fever, as originally proposed by NIMMANNITYA et al. (1969):

Grade I   Fever accompanied by nonspecific constitutional symptoms, with a positive tourniquet test as the only hemorrhagic manifestation.

Grade II   Fever and skin hemorrhage or other bleeding such as epistaxis or gum bleeding.

Grade III   Circulatory failure manifested by rapid, weak pulse with narrowing of the pulse pressure (< 20 mm Hg) or hypotension.

Grade IV   Moribund patients with undetectable blood pressure and pulse.

Carefully documented studies on the incidence and nature of dengue and chikungunya virus infections in children occurring between 1962 and 1964 in Thailand were published by HALSTEAD and his coworkers (NIMMANNITYA et al., 1969; HALSTEAD et al., 1969a—d). They estimated that, in 1962 alone, between 181,000 and 287,000 dengue illnesses and between 44,000 and 70,000 chikungunya illnesses were seen in ambulatory patients (HALSTEAD et al., 1969c). During their three-year study, 10,194 patients with "HF" were hospitalized, and the authors assumed that at least 80% of these were infected with dengue virus. Five-hundred-fifty-nine of the patients died, and the overall mortality rate has been variously estimated to range from 5 to 15%. The overwhelming majority of patients hospitalized with symptoms of HF were children under 15 years of age.

A group of 639 children were selected for detailed study of clinical and etiological parameters (NIMMANNITYA et al., 1969). Of these 523 were identified as having dengue HF, and 202 were classified as Grades III and IV (shock). The death rate among the shock patients was 10%. The age distribution of dengue and chikungunya

patients in this special study is shown in Fig. 30 (Fig. 5 from NIMMANNITYA *et al.*).
It is clear that there were two peak age groups affected by HF: (1) infants under
1 year; (2) children between 3 and 6 (modal 4) years of age. A more detailed
analysis of incidence in infants during the first year of life demonstrated that
most of them acquired HF during the second half, *i.e.*, after 6 months of age
(see below) (HALSTEAD *et al.*, 1969c).

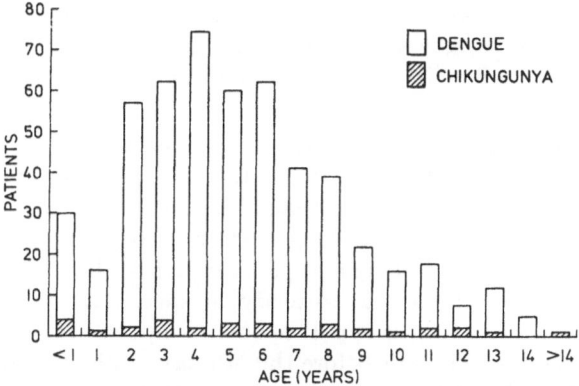

Fig. 30. Graph showing age distribution among 523 patients with confirmed dengue
and 30 with confirmed chikungunya virus infection with a diagnosis at discharge of
hemorrhagic fever. CH and CRC Study, 1962—1964. From NIMMANNITYA *et al.* (1969)
With permission of the authors and the American Journal of Tropical Medicine
and Hygiene

Clinical laboratory findings in DHF and DSS differed from those in uncomplicated "classical" dengue fever in several respects (NIMMANNITYA *et al.*, 1969; HALSTEAD
et al., 1970c). Patients *not in shock* had a near normal leukocyte count and no
consistent lymphocytosis. Their thrombocyte counts were only slightly and tran-
siently lowered. Some of these patients had hypoproteinemia, elevated serum
transaminase levels, and evidence of hemoconcentration. Patients *in shock*
exhibited thrombocytopenia and other evidence of hemoconcentration and
unbalanced hemostasis with far greater frequency and intensity.

Pathological findings have been discussed extensively in the various symposia
and monographs listed above. A series of 100 autopsy cases was described by
BHAMARAPRAVATI *et al.* (1967). In general, the picture is one of "non-specific"
damage to blood vessels without necrosis, degenerative changes, or inflammation.
Petechial or more extensive hemorrhages are evident in various organs, and there
is increased fluid in the body cavities. The liver may show degenerative foci
resembling those found in yellow fever, including Councilman bodies (cf. HOTTA,
1969).

3. Virological and Serological Findings

As already indicated, DHF and DSS have been seen in large-scale epidemic
form in those parts of South and Southeast Asia in which two or more dengue
serotypes are endemic. The most comprehensive clinical, epidemiological, virological,
and serological data were collected and analyzed over a number of years (1958

to 1964) in Bangkok, Thailand, by HALSTEAD and his colleagues (NIMMANNITYA
et al., 1969; HALSTEAD et al., 1969a—d, HALSTEAD, 1970, 1971; HALSTEAD et al.,
1970a—c; FISCHER and HALSTEAD, 1970; NISALAK et al., 1970).

To summarize briefly: (a) All four dengue serotypes were present endemically;
(b) the viruses were transmitted almost exclusively by A. aegypti; (c) the annual
infection rate of the native population was estimated at 15%, considerably lower
for temporary nonindigenous white residents; (d) the age-related incidence of
DHF and DSS showed two peaks: one in infants 7—8 months of age who were
born of mothers with dengue antibodies and who gave a *primary* response, the
second in children 2 to 8 years of age (modal age 4 years) who gave a secondary
immune response.

Primary and secondary responses were defined as follows: ··*Primary* infection
with dengue virus was assumed: (1) if acute-phase plasma through the fourth
day of illness contained no detectable dengue HI antibody at a 1:20 dilution and
14- to 21-day specimens contained dengue HI antibody at dilutions of 1:1280
or below, or (2) if a monotypic dengue type 1 through 4 CF response was observed
in patients with undetectable CF antibody in specimens obtained before the
7th day of disease. *Secondary* group B arbovirus infection was assumed: (1) if
plasma specimens obtained on or before the 4th day of illness contained HI antibody at a 1:20 or higher dilution, or (2) if 14- to 21-day specimens contained HI
antibody at dilutions of 1:2560 or higher, or (3) if CF antibody to two or more
dengue antigens was present in plasma obtained during the first 7 days of illness."
(NIMMANNITYA et al., 1969.) It should be noted that, among randomly selected
patients with confirmed secondary dengue, a high proportion displayed HI antibody titers of $\geq 1:20,480$ quite early after onset (Fig. 31). The broadly cross-
reactive type of HI and CF response to all 4 dengue serotypes is illustrated in
RUSSELL (1970) (Table 25). In contrast to primary dengue infections in which the
usual pattern is initial production of 19S IgM antiviral antibodies followed by
that of 7S IgG, the rapid response to secondary infection is almost entirely 7S in
nature (RUSSELL et al., 1969; RUSSELL, 1971).

Table 25. *Examples of typical serologic responses to dengue infection in Thai children*

Type infection	Day of illness	Hemagglutination-inhibition				Complement fixation			
		D-1	D-2	D-3	D-4	D-1	D-2	D-3	D-4
Primary[a]	3	<10[c]	<10	<10	<10	<4[d]	<4	<4	<4
	16	20	20	40	320	<4	4	<4	8
Secondary[b]	3	40	160	80	80	4	16	4	8
	10	>10,240	>10,240	>10,240	>10,240	128	256	256	512

[a] Dengue-4 infection; mild illness.
[b] Dengue-4 infection; serotype of previous infection unknown. Severe illness with shock.
[c] Reciprocal titer vs. 8 U of antigen.
[d] Reciprocal titer vs. 2 U of antigen with 2 exact U of complement.

From RUSSELL (1970). With permission of the author and Grune & Stratton, Inc.,
New York, representing Schwabe and Co., Basel-Stuttgart, publishers.

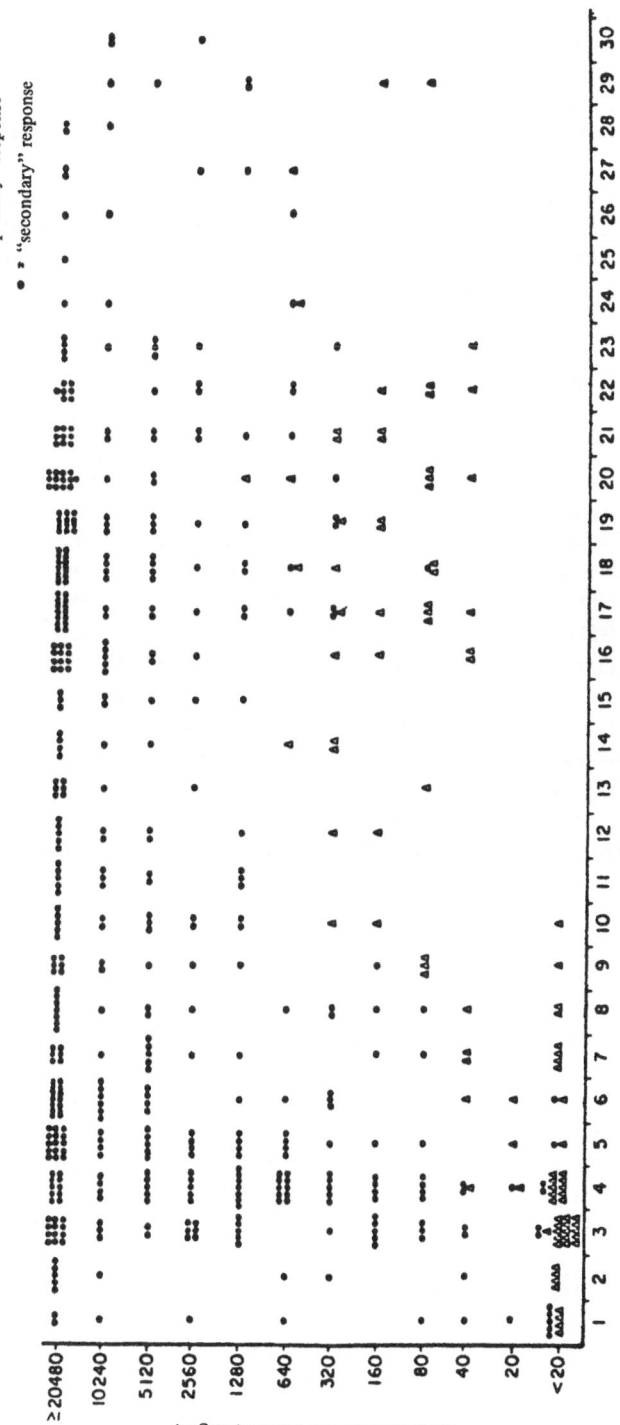

Fig. 31. Schema of HI-antibody titers to dengue-1 antigen in a random selection of 50% of patients with confirmed dengue infection and a diagnosis at discharge of hemorrhagic fever. Antibody responses considered "primary" and "secondary" are indicated. CH and CRC Study, 1962—1964. From NIMMANNITYA et al. (1969)

With permission of the authors and the American Journal of Tropical Medicine and Hygiene

Generally, the frequency of successful virus isolation from patients with DHF or DSS is much lower then from those with primary dengue (NIMMANNITYA et al.. 1969; HALSTEAD et al., 1970c). This is obviously related to the accelerated and extremely high antibody response in secondary infections. and it has been suggested that virus recovery may be facilitated by techniques that dissociate virions and antibody. such as the "delayed plaque technique" of YUILL et al. (1968). HALSTEAD et al. (1970c) in their study of 523 children with serologically confirmed dengue (including 71 with primary dengue immune responses) hospitalized in Bangkok between 1962 and 1964 found that only 89 (15%) yielded virus at any time during the acute phase. Large-scale epidemiological investigations during this period indicated that dengue-1, -2, and -3 viruses were about evenly distributed in mosquito vectors and in patients with primary dengue. Nevertheless, among those with secondary infection dengue-2 virus was recovered significantly more often than the other serotypes. The rate of virus isolation was inversely related to the grade of severity, and NISALAK et al. (1970) were able to recover only 4 virus isolates from 103 postmortem sera and 2 additional ones from 523 organs obtained at autopsy from 98 fatal cases of DSS.

A particularly instructive study, confirming in all essentials the findings in Bangkok, was that of two consecutive outbreaks of DHF on Koh Samui, a small island in the Gulf of Thailand (WINTER et al., 1968, 1969, 1971; RUSSELL et al., 1968; SMITH et al., 1971).

Another comprehensive analysis of 55 cases was carried out in 1971 in connection with a collaborative study of pathogenetic mechanisms in DHF (WHO Report, 1973; see below). Of the 55 cases, 2 were primary infections of infants <6 months of age whose mothers possessed dengue HI antibodies; 2 were fatal cases; of the remaining 51 secondary infections, 18 were clinically grade I or II, 23 grade III, 10 grade IV. Viruses were isolated from only 9 of the 55 patients (8 type 2, 1 type 1). Virus recovery appeared to be favored by obtaining early blood specimens (<4 days after onset) which had relatively low HI antibody titers ($<^1/_{160}$ in the WHO study).

4. Immunopathology of Secondary Dengue

Because of the overwhelming evidence suggesting the preponderant role of secondary dengue infection and of accompanying immunopathological mechanisms in the pathogenesis of HF and, especially, DSS, several authors have investigated in depth the levels of complement components and other serum factors as a measure of complement consumption and/or pharmacologically active mediators of vascular damage. These individual efforts (e.g., HALSTEAD et al., 1967; WINTER et al., 1968; RUSSELL et al., 1969; RUSSELL, 1970, 1971; RUSSELL and BRANDT, 1973) culminated in a systematic collaborative study of selected pediatric patients with DHF and DSS hospitalized in July—September 1971 in Bangkok (BOKISCH et al., 1973; WHO Report, 1973). Of an estimated total of over 500 hospitalized patients. 55 with virological or serological evidence of dengue were selected for detailed analysis (Table 26), along with various suitable non-dengue control patients. At the time of this outbreak, at least three dengue serotypes (-1, -2, -3) were present in Bangkok. As mentioned above, from only 9 of the 55 patients was virus isolated. Serological responses of the secondary type were seen in 51/55 patients (Fig. 32).

Two infants <6 months old showed a primary response, but the mothers of both had dengue HI antibody. The remaining two were fatal cases from whom suitable serum specimens were not available.

In confirmation of earlier reports by RUSSELL (1971; RUSSELL and BRANDT, 1973), it was found that various complement components were markedly depressed in patients with DSS. In particular, the degree of depression of C3 was correlated

Table 26. *Numbers of primary and secondary HI antibody responses in 55 patients, according to the severity of the disease*

Grade(s) of disease	Primary infection (convalescent titer < 640)	Secondary infection (convalescent titer > 640)	Unclassifiable
I and II	1	18	0
III	0	23	0
IV	1	10	2
Totals	2[a]	51	2[b]

[a] Both infants <6 months of age.
[b] Both deaths. Convalescent serum not available.

From WHO Report (1973). With permission of the Office of Publications, World Health Organization.

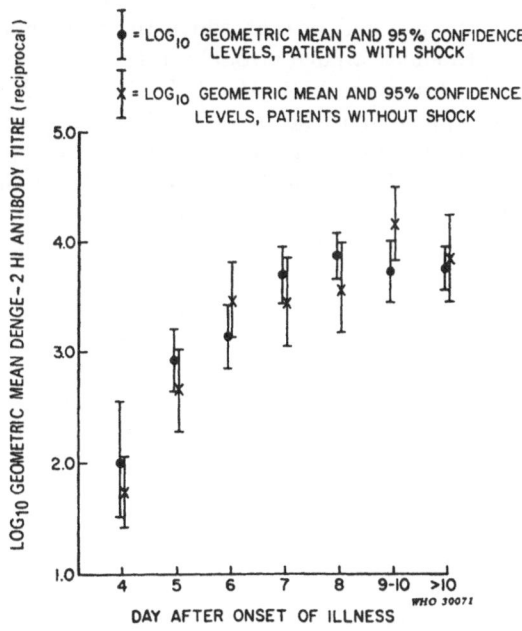

Fig. 32. Dengue-2 HI antibody titers following onset of disease in patients with and without shock. From WHO Report (1973)
With permission of the Office of Publications, World Health Organization

with the severity of disease, but in grade III and IV patients C3 proactivator
(C3PA), C4, and C5 were also greatly reduced. $C1_q$, $C1_s$, C6, as well as fibrinogen
were slightly depressed in the most severe forms, transferrin about equally and
very slightly in all grades (Fig. 33). The greatest mean depression of C3, C3PA,
C4, as well as of fibrinogen and of platelet counts occurred at onset and during
the first 2 days after onset of shock.

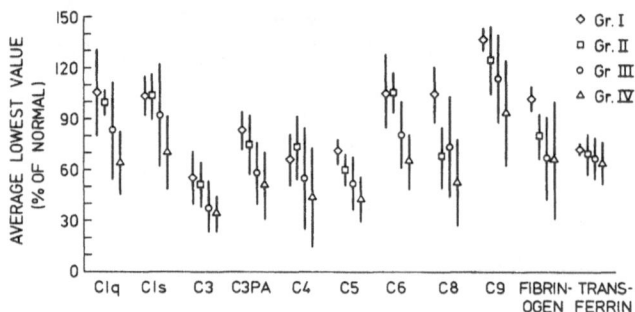

Fig. 33. Mean lowest values (± 1 standard deviation) of various complement proteins
and fibrinogen from 55 individuals with serologically established dengue infection.
Transferrin was measured as a noncomplement protein control. From WHO Report
(1973)
With permission of the Office of Publications, World Health Organization

It was concluded that the rapid rate at which the complement components
decreased in patients with shock argued strongly in favor of complement activation and consumption. Moreover, both the "classical" and the "alternate"
pathways of activation appeared to be involved. Together with the fact that
hemorrhagic disease and shock are characteristically seen when virus and antibody
are present simultaneously in the patient, these findings favor the view that one
of the underlying mechanisms is intravascular antigen-antibody complex formation (see Fig. 34). To quote (WHO Report, 1973): "What might be the pathological
consequences of a massive activation of complement? Activation of C3 and 5 is
accompanied by dissociation of low molecular weight peptides called C3a and 5a,
which have the capacity to release histamine and are very potent permeability
increasing factors ..." and "A plausible working hypothesis is ... (that), as a
result of dengue virus infection in a patient with pre-existing antibody, an immunopathological process possibly involving immune complexes or another $C1_q$ reactive
substance leads to massive complement activation ... (This) is accompanied by
the liberation of vasoactive peptides (anaphylatoxins) and by initiation of intravascular blood coagulation, followed by partial, often severe, depletion of plasma
complement components owing to the rapid removal of complement reaction
products from the circulation. The simultaneous activation of proteolytic enzymes
of the complement, coagulation, and possibly the kinin, systems may be expected
to consume plasma enzyme inhibitors. Partial depletion of these inhibitors may
result in an imbalance between activated enzymes and inhibitors and thus produce
increased vascular permeability and shock."

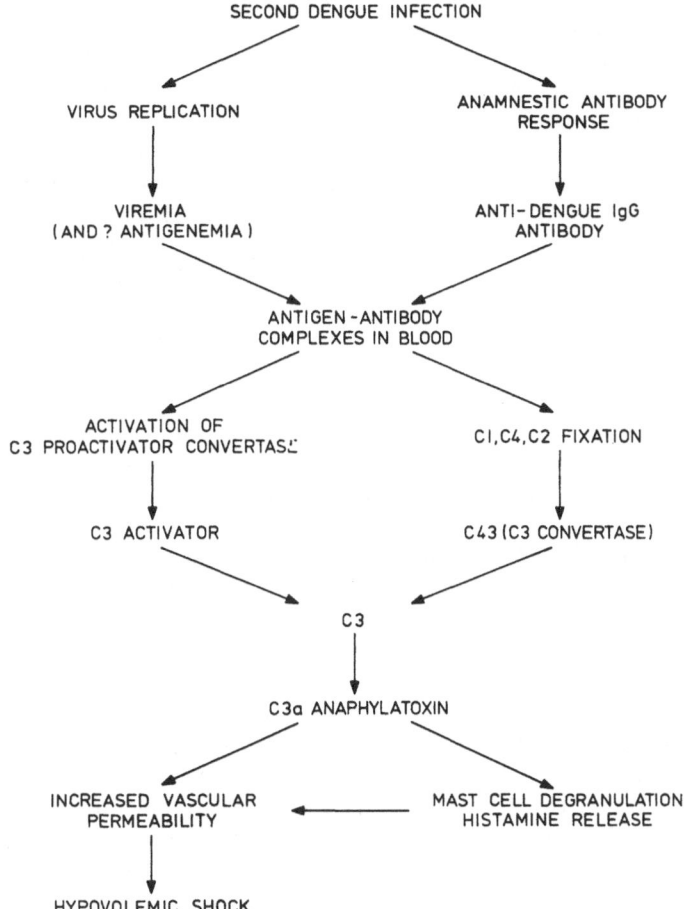

Fig. 34. Current concept of the immunopathologic mechanisms causing the dengue shock syndrome. From RUSSELL and BRANDT (1973) With permission of the authors and Academic Press, Inc., New York

The evidence presented in support of this working hypothesis is persuasive indeed. It should be stressed, however, that its statement, as quoted, is too broad and requires several qualifications. It is *not* true that DHF and DSS occur "as a result of dengue virus infection in a patient with pre-existing antibody": (1) We have discussed (see Section X. B. 3. on Immunity) that primary dengue infection leads to solid (and probably life-long) protection against reinfection with homotypic virus and that resistance to heterotypic strains in male adults is evanescent and gradually diminishes over a period of about 9 months. Antibodies persist, but there is no associated predisposition to DHF or DSS. (2) WISSEMAN et al. (1966) as well as others (see Section XI) have shown that mere presence of dengue cross-neutralizing antibodies resulting from previous experience with Japanese encephalitis virus and/or YF vaccination failed to diminish or modify the clinical reaction of adult subjects to experimental infection with dengue virus. (3) In several geographic areas in which epidemic incursions by different dengue serotypes were separated by several years (*e.g.*, the Caribbean, see Figs. 1—3), no DHF or DSS have been seen, despite the high incidence of pre-existing heterotypic antibodies at the time of the second epidemic (cf. EHRENKRANZ *et al.*, 1971). (4) Although the frequency of occurrence of HI antibody to just one of the four dengue serotypes (-1) in a large population sample in Bangkok was 80—90% at age 15 years or higher (HALSTEAD *et al.*, 1969c), the occurrence of DHF or DSS peaked at 2 to 8 years of age and was virtually zero at more than 14 years of age (NIMMANNITYA *et al.*, 1969). (5) Similarly, although newborn babies in that population can acquire dengue infection at any time during the first year of life, the incidence ot DHF and DSS are characteristically highest in those who acquire their infection in the second half, when transplacentally acquired maternal antibodies have declined significantly (HALSTEAD, 1971).

Hence the working hypothesis must explain (1) the *age-specific* incidence of DHF, (2) the obvious requirement for *sequential infections* with *two different* dengue serotypes, (3) the probability that DHF is precipitated by a *second* infection with a dengue serotype other than that causing the first one but that subsequent additional infections (with yet other types) appear to involve no risk for a second attack of DHF, (4) the apparent failure of group B togaviruses other than dengue viruses to "sensitize" individuals in such a way that DHF occurs, (5) the absence of DHF in certain areas known to have supported extensive epidemics caused by different dengue serotypes.

The key to meeting these qualifying conditions seems to lie in the fact that DHF and DSS have thus far been limited to South and Southeast Asian countries where all four or at least three dengue serotypes are highly and about equally prevalent and where the vector density is so high that the annual transmission rate has been estimated as high as 15% of the indigenous human population. The mathematical model of FISCHER and HALSTEAD (1970) based on these statistics and HALSTEAD's (1970) general discussion would suggest that a crucial element is reinfection at a time when the dengue subgroup cross-reactive antibodies result- ing from first infection (or from transplacental transfer) have decreased to a threshold level low enough to allow virus replication and the formation of antigen- antibody complexes at some critical stage of the disease.

The nature and location of these complexes remain to be elucidated (WHO Report, 1973; RUSSELL and BRANDT, 1973). One can speculate, however, that (a) the group B-cross-reactive antigens (presumably nucleocapsid and the envelope glycoprotein) are probably not involved since antibodies to non-dengue flaviviruses do not seem to predispose to DHF or DSS; (b) the type-specific antigen (presumably associated with envelope glycoprotein VP-3) does not seem to be responsible since homotypic reinfection does not lead to DHF or DSS; (c) the SCF antigen (see Section VI. E. 4.) does not seem to be responsible (RUSSELL and BRANDT, 1973). The most likely candidates for the responsible antigens would be virion- or cell- associated dengue subgroup-specific proteins, but the nature of these has not yet been clearly identified (see Section VI. E. 2.).

With regard to the fact that DHF and DSS are essentially limited to children, this seems logical in view of the immunological constraints just discussed combined

with the extraordinarily high transmission rates existing in the indigenous population. Thus, an individual is at high risk of acquiring a second infection with a
different serotype at a critical time after the first (sensitizing) infection. The critical
time interval has been estimated by HALSTEAD (1970) to be somewhere between
3 months and 5 years. With an estimated annual transmission rate of 15%, this
requirement is most likely to be met during childhood. It is, of course, possible
that age-related physiological factors may play an additional and equally important role.

The mathematical models constructed by FISCHER and HALSTEAD (1970)
from age-specific hospitalization rates in Bangkok "fit predicted sequential
infection rates only when it was assumed that the second (but not the third or
fourth) dengue infection elicited a hypersensitivity reaction" (HALSTEAD, 1970).
Effective protection against antigen-antibody complex formation would indeed
be expected in hyperimmune patients who possess broadly cross-reactive antibodies as a result of two sequential infections with different serotypes (see Table 25).

Finally, there remain several other questions with regard to the hemorrhagic
fever problem to which no or only fragmentary answers are now available:
(1) Why is it that dengue-2 virus appears to be isolated from (and associated with?)
DHF and DSS more frequently than the other serotypes? HALSTEAD (1970)
suggests that this may be related to its being a "better" antigen (HALSTEAD et al.,
1970a), its greater replicative capacity, or its more frequent neutralization by
heterotypic antisera (HALSTEAD and SIMASTHIEN, 1970). (2) Are there racial,
ethnic, or economic factors which predispose to DHF or DSS? Apparently not:
exhaustive epidemiological analyses by HALSTEAD et al. (1969c) show that dengue-
related hospitalization rates (taken as a valid measure of clinical complications)
for Thai and Chinese resident children were alike in proportion to the respective
overall infection rates with dengue viruses. Other races and ethnic groups have
been involved in the Philippine Islands, India, Ceylon, presumably with similar
proportionalities. In Thailand, the overall dengue infection rate among non-
indigenous white populations is far lower than among the native population, and
this is correlated with much lower rate of exposure to Aedes aegypti, effective
mosquito control, and absence of water storage facilities suitable for breeding
(HALSTEAD et al., 1969b). Nevertheless, at least one fatal case of DSS in an American child has been reported (RUSSELL et al., 1967). (3) Outbreaks on Pacific
Islands of dengue have been reported (MOREAU et al., 1973; BARNES and ROSEN,
1974) which were characterized by severe hemorrhagic manifestations and shock
(some fatal) but did not fit the historical-epidemiological patterns of DHF and
DSS in highly endemic countries of Southeast Asia: not all infections seem to have
been secondary, and those that were, were separated from last previous exposure
by as much as 25 years; there was no age-specific difference in incidence; the
time of onset and the nature and distribution of hemorrhagic lesions or shock
differed from those described elsewhere. Therefore ROSEN and coworkers have
disputed the validity of the "second infection" hypothesis championed by
HALSTEAD, RUSSELL, and their associates. Earlier, HAMMON (1973) had also
raised questions about the compatibility of all observations with a unified concept
of immunopathological mechanisms. Granting that the episodes described by
ROSEN's group were indeed cases of hemorrhagic dengue uncomplicated by

unrelated underlying or superimposed illnesses, it seems entirely feasible that in
such insular outbreaks a variant form of dengue may arise in which the patho-
gnomonic minor hemorrhagic lesions (petechiae) are exacerbated and extended
in severity (see Section X. B. for discussion of the variable incidence of petechiae
in natural and experimental infections). These lesions occur characteristically
late, *i.e.*, at the end of or after the febrile acute phase of illness. This circumstance
suggests that petechiae may be a minimal manifestation of the same basic immunopathological process (antigen excess at the time of incipient antibody formation,
leading to immune complex formation etc.) postulated for DHF and DSS in the
"second infection" hypothesis. The occurrence of more severe hemorrhagic *primary*
disease in circumscribed epidemics or in rare individual victims during large-scale
epidemics could conceivably be due to special viral variants, to defects in immune
response, in short, to any variable that would lead to an effective modification
of antigen/antibody ratios at a critical stage in the disease. Moreover, since the
nature of the antigen(s) and antibody(ies) reacting in immune complexes has not
been identified, it remains possible that they may involve not only virus-specific
reactants but also cross-reactive antigen(s) to which certain patients have been
sensitized by some stimulus other than a group B togavirus infection.

XI. Immunization

A. Anamnestic Immune Responses in Sequential Infections With Dengue and Other Group B Togaviruses

1. Results With Members of the Dengue Subgroup

Acceptance of the "second infection" hypothesis as a valid explanation of the
pathogenesis of DHF and DSS has obvious implications for the problem of
immunization against dengue fever. The question is whether possession of cross-
reactive antibodies resulting from vaccination may, at least in some individuals,
predispose to aggravated illness upon subsequent infection. The notion that such
antibodies are not necessarily protective is supported by field and experimental
observations going back to SILER *et al.* (1926) and SIMMONS *et al.* (1931). In more
specific terms, SABIN's (1952a) experiments in adult human volunteers with types
1 and 2 showed that cross protection was effective for only about 2 months, then
waned until after 9 months heterologous reinfection produced definite, though
still modified, illness. The case described by CAREY *et al.* (1965) in which two
episodes of disease, one caused by type 4, the other by type 1, occurred 1 year
apart in the same individual, has already been discussed.

   In these situations, as well as in others perhaps less systematically documented,
antibodies reacting with the second infecting virus were either present at the time
of reinfection or were produced rapidly and in copious amounts, indicating an
anamnestic response. In either case, they did not confer complete protection,
clearly suggesting that something more (or other) than cross-reactive antibody
is required for an effective immune mechanism and that this is as true in adults
as it is in children who are subject to the further complication of DHF and DSS.

   The validity of this conclusion is supported by experiments on monkeys.
WHITEHEAD *et al.* (1970) subjected gibbons *(Hylobates lar)* to sequential infections

with the four dengue serotypes in varying combinations. They found that animals first infected with dengue-2, -3, or -4 viruses, all of which induced viremia, developed viremia again when challenged 12 weeks later with types 1, 2, or 4, but not with type 3. Heterologous reinfection of gibbons first infected with dengue-1 virus failed to induce viremia. Even third viremias were induced when the infection sequence was dengue-2-4-1. In all instances leading to second or third viremia, neutralizing and HI antibodies to the challenge virus were present at the time of challenge. Very similar findings were reported by SCHERER et al. (1972) who used small New World monkeys (marmosets and squirrel monkeys) rather than gibbons.

More extensive comparative studies by HALSTEAD and coworkers (HALSTEAD et al., 1973a, c, d; HALSTEAD and PALUMBO, 1973; MARCHETTE et al., 1973) involved primary and secondary infections at different m. o. i.'s of rhesus monkeys and included detailed analysis of the distribution of virus in various tissues, serological response, and "clinical laboratory" data. All monkeys were free of detectable dengue antibodies prior to first infection, developed viremia beginning 1 to >7 days after inoculation of 5×10^3—5×10^5 pfu (mean day of onset 3.15 for dengue-1, 3.04 for -2, 4.66 for -3, 3.16 for -4) which lasted several days (means 4.58, 3.95, 1.83, 3.64 days for the viruses in numerical order); all exhibited HI and CF antibody responses by 21 days p.i. which cross-reacted with all four dengue-types as well as with five other flaviviruses. Significant percentages of the test animals had leukopenia and relative lymphocytosis (especially in dengue-2 infections). No major abnormalities occurred in platelet counts, hematocrit, total serum protein, or prothrombin time. Complement levels showed a tendency to be increased.

One-hundred-eighteen monkeys were challenged at intervals ranging from 2 to 26 weeks after the primary infection. Animals challenged with dengue-2 or -4 at 2 weeks after primary type 1 infection did not develop viremia; nor did those challenged with dengue-3 at *any* interval after primary heterotypic infection. In the other combinations, viremia was not ablated, except in some cases of challenge with dengue-4. In those that did develop viremia after challenge with dengue-1 or -4, the onset was delayed, duration shorter, and peak titers tended to be lower compared with corresponding primary infections.

In contrast, peak titers in secondary dengue-2 viremia tended to be significantly higher than in primary infection, and this was associated in several animals with mild thrombocytopenia and, perhaps of greatest interest, with an early decrease in total complement. One monkey whose course after infection with dengue-4, followed 3 months later by dengue-2, was documented in detail by HALSTEAD et al. (1973d) is of special interest because the "abnormalities recapitulate most of the important laboratory findings observed in DSS in man". This was also true for the antibody responses in all heterotypically challenged animals.

Especially revealing were the assays for virus in various tissues of monkeys after primary or secondary infections (MARCHETTE et al., 1973). Briefly, virus was rapidly disseminated from the site of subcutaneous inoculation to the draining lymphnodes and thence to lymphatic tissues throughout the body. In primary as well as secondary infection, two to three days after onset of viremia and for about 3 days after viremia, virus was also found in various skin sites, in the respiratory tract, in other tissues and in circulating leukocytes. Remarkably, this study suggests that the rate of virus recovery from various tissues may be higher in secondary heterotypic than in primary infection.

It must be pointed out that experiments on monkeys provide a useful but only partially valid model for the situation in man: (1) dengue viruses do not cause manifest clinical illness in monkeys; (2) the data on viremia and virus distribution in monkeys were obtained during periods following inoculations which would, in man, correspond to or overlap into the incubation period. Comparable data for man are therefore not available, and the relevance of such early events to variable clinical responses of naturally infected patients remains to be demonstrated; (3) the virus doses inoculated subcutaneously in secondary infections may have been considerably larger than those transmitted by mosquitoes in nature.

Nevertheless, the experiments on monkeys reinforce the principle that effective protection against heterotypic second dengue infections must require factors other than preexisting antibodies or the capacity to respond anamnestically.

Their provocative findings on sequential infections led HALSTEAD et al. (1973 b) to a study of the effects of sensitization of monkey leukocytes by prior infection of the donor animal with dengue-4 virus. In preliminary experiments, they found a remarkable increase in lymphoblast transformation and viral yield following in vitro challenge with dengue-2.

The question of whether specific sensitization by a heterologous dengue virus was required, or whether non-specific blast transformation (e.g., by phytohemagglutinin) could likewise stimulate enhanced viral replication was not unequivocally resolved. However, a more recent report by the same group (SUNG et al., 1975) describes dengue virus replication, SCF antigen production, and establishment of persistent dengue infection in continuous human lymphoblastoid cell lines derived from Burkitt lymphoma or leukemia patients. Thus, while it could be said that these cells seem simply to share with other multiplying human cells the capacity to support replication of dengue viruses (cf. Section V), there is something singularly intriguing about the fact that antigenic challenge of appropriately sensitized leukocytes is one way to bring about blast transformation. In other words, even if specific sensitization is not required for enhancement of in vitro viral growth, it may in fact be the only biologically relevant mechanism operating in vivo. The implications would be that, in an immune host,

(1) homologous challenge virus would be neutralized and destroyed,

(2) heterologous challenge virus may be damaged by cross-reactive antibody of low avidity or only partial specificity, but not prevented from initiating infection of circulating sensitized leukocytes;

(3) infection of the latter may then lead to cell division, viral replication and antigen production, and resultant dissemination throughout the organism as well as disease production;

(4) this sequence of events might be further complicated, under conditions favoring immune complex formation (see Section X), by hemorrhagic diathesis and shock.

Further confirmation and extension of this exciting work is basic not only to an understanding of pathogenetic principles but also to the rational development of immunization schemes. For example, it has already been suggested by the work of HALSTEAD et al. (1973a) and of HALSTEAD and PALUMBO (1973) that protection of rhesus monkeys against all four dengue serotypes is more effectively produced by simultaneous immunization with 3 or 4 types than by their sequential administration. In terms of the preceding discussion, this would make sense because the simultaneous dosage would presumably by-pass the stage of sensitization of circulating leukocytes. On the other hand, simultaneous administration (either of mixtures or by inoculation at separate sites) would entail the risk of interference by one with replication of other virus(es) to adequately immunogenic levels and thus necessitate extremely careful adjustment of dosage.

2. Results With Dengue and Other Flaviviruses

In view of the result obtained with virus sequences within the dengue subgroup, it is not surprising that experimental and epidemiological observations have consistently failed to reveal significant reciprocal protection between dengue and other group B togaviruses. For example, the effects of yellow fever 17 D vaccination on dengue infection were studied in human volunteers by SABIN (1952a) and summarized by him as follows: "(1) When dengue virus, in amounts of 10 to 1 million human MID, was inoculated *simultaneously* with, or *3 days after*, yellow fever vaccine, the onset of dengue was delayed for 3 to 6 days, and the resulting disease was milder and of shorter duration. (2) When dengue virus was injected *1 week* after the yellow fever vaccine, the incubation period was unaffected, but the resulting disease was milder and of shorter duration. (3) When infection with dengue virus (either by the bites of infected mosquitoes or the inoculation of 10 human M.I.D. of infectious serum) was postponed for *5 weeks* after the yellow fever vaccine, neither the incubation period nor the duration or severity of the resulting dengue were modified."

These results suggest the operation of an evanescent interfering effect by YFV on dengue virus. In a follow-up, WISSEMAN et al. (1966) found that experimental subjects who had either had a subclinical infection with Japanese encephalitis virus or been vaccinated against yellow fever 30 days prior to challenge with dengue-1 virus, *or both*, developed typical and unmodified dengue fever. This included viremia, even in those individuals whose undiluted serum, collected about the time of onset, cross-neutralized dengue-1 virus. Similarly, HALSTEAD et al. (1969b) found that previous YF vaccination had no effect on the extent or duration of dengue viremia.

GROSSBERG and SCHERER (1958) reported that accidental dengue-1 infection of a laboratory worker who had antibodies to JEV as a result of naturally acquired inapparent infection developed unmodified clinical illness. It should be mentioned again that, in the study of Japanese encephalitis in Chiangmai Valley, Thailand (GROSSMAN et al., 1974), sera of U.S. servicemen with histories of YF vaccination or of natives presumed to have had dengue cross-reacted broadly; but the IgM fractions were monospecific for JEV (EDELMAN et al., 1973).

Conversely, it has been suggested that prior experience with dengue may have a marginal attenuating effect on the incidence of clinical encephalitis following exposure to JE (HAMMON et al., 1966; GROSSMAN et al., 1974) or SLE viruses

(BOND and HAMMON, 1970); these retrospective seroepidemiological analyses are somewhat tenuous and would require extensive corroboration.

Experiments by TARR and HAMMON (1974) do provide some interesting support for such a relationship between dengue-2 hyperimmunization of mice followed 4—20 weeks later by subcutaneous challenges with JE or SLE viruses. Significant resistance to the heterologous viruses was observed even when the immunosuppressant cyclophosphamide was administered 24 hours after the challenge dose.

Against this background, PRICE and his associates have devoted exhaustive efforts and have published numerous papers on the use of various immunization sequences with which to achieve protection of experimental animals against many group B togaviruses, including the four dengue serotypes (see PRICE *et al.*, 1973a, b, for comprehensive citation of references). Briefly, their studies culminated in the elaboration of a sequential immunization procedure which protected spider monkeys against 20 viruses in terms of across-the-board HI and neutralizing antibody, suppression of viremia (13 viruses tested), and (where applicable) lesions produced in the central nervous system. The vaccines, injected intramuscularly, were all suckling mouse brain homogenates. The schedule was (1) 17D YF virus. 10^5 LD_{50}; (2) Langat E5 virus, 3×10^6 LD_{50}, 1 month later; (3) dengue-2, New Guinea C. 3×10^6 LD_{50}, 1 month later. Challenge viruses were administered subcutaneously four months after the last vaccination, *i.e.*, at a time when challenge of a dengue-immunized human being with a heterotypic dengue virus may reveal complete or partial protection.

Although PRICE *et al.* (1973a) recommend exploration of their sequential scheme for possible use in man. there are compelling reasons for caution. These are discussed below.

B. Dengue Vaccines for Use in Man

This section will present a discussion of the status of dengue vaccines and of factors that might be considered as guidelines for future developments.

During World War II it was conclusively demonstrated that continued intracerebral passage of dengue-1 virus in mice was associated with the changes in viral properties discussed in Chapter IX. These changes included attenuation of human pathogenicity and thus provided the basis for successful vaccination of human volunteers with the Mochizuki (KIMURA and HOTTA, 1944; cf. HOTTA 1965, 1969) and Hawai strains (SABIN and SCHLESINGER, 1945; cf. SABIN, 1952a). "Success" in these early experiments was measured in terms of complete protection against reinfection with homologous unmodified virus, either by injection or by mosquito transmission. The virus in the mouse brain vaccines induced rashes in most of the inoculated volunteers, but usually other signs or symptoms were absent or trivial (low-grade fever of 1—2 days' duration). Similar reactions were induced with the Hawaii strain grown in chick embryos (SCHLESINGER, 1951).

Dengue-2 virus was shown to undergo a similar modification upon passage in mice (SCHLESINGER and FRANKEL, 1952a; SABIN, 1955; SCHLESINGER *et al.*, 1956). For further details regarding the characteristics of human reactions to these vaccines and tests for immunity the cited references should be consulted. In the present context, it suffices to say that these experiments indicated the feasibility of developing attenuated virus stocks as well as their immunogenic potency.

On the other hand, it had also been demonstrated that inactivation of un-modified (human or mosquito) virus by formalin or UV irradiation (SABIN, 1952 a) or of early mouse passage ("unmodified") dengue-1 virus by ox bile (HOTTA, 1954; cf. HOTTA, 1965, 1969) led to total or partial loss of immunogenicity.

Of more important concern, in light of current knowledge about dengue viruses, are the questions raised in the following paragraphs. Although definitive answers to these questions cannot be given, the technology for dealing with many of them is available.

(1) *Is attenuation by intracerebral passages in mice a sound basis for vaccine development?*

As discussed in detail in Section IX. A., random viral stocks derived from continuing intracerebral passages in mice acquire in increasing degree of neuro-virulence—not only for mice but also for chick embryos (SCHLESINGER, 1951), hamsters (MEIKLEJOHN et al., 1952 b), and monkeys (SABIN, 1955). Thus, the use of such preparations in man, even in partially purified form, entails the risks of contamination with neural tissue components as well as of potential human neurovirulence. Although no indications of neurological complications accompanied the vaccination trials referred to above, the total number of people involved was far too small to be sanguine about this risk, particularly if children were to be vaccinated [see item (5)]. This problem was recognized by PRICE et al. (1973 b), and they sought to solve it by subjecting dengue-2 virus (New Guinea C strain, 26th mouse brain passage) to 129 continued serial passages and final plaque purifica-tion in African green monkey kidney cell cultures. This procedure was reported to result in reduction of neurovirulence for monkeys (but apparently not for mice) as judged by clinical signs and histological lesions after intracerebral or intraspinal inoculation. It was this variant which, after a further series of passages in suckling mice, was used in the sequential immunization schemes discussed in the preceding section. Clearly, the manner in which this variant was derived and tested for stability would be too haphazard for practical usefulness. It seems clear that a deliberate search for suitable mutants lacking neurovirulence and other undesirable traits must be based on the establishment of reliable covariant functions more easily and meaningfully tested than by inoculation of a few monkeys.

Of possible interest in this connection is the dengue-1 (Hawaii) vaccine ("MD-1 variant") derived by WISSEMAN et al. (1963) from the 18th passage of SABIN and SCHLESINGER's original series by 13—14 additional suckling mouse passages. It produced no rash or other clinical manifestations in human volunteers. Yet it was fully effective both in terms of antibody response and protection against challenge with unmodified virus (WISSEMAN et al., 1963; WISSEMAN, 1966). Indeed, this is the only dengue vaccine that has been tested under field conditions during the Puerto Rico epidemic of 1963 (WISSEMAN, 1966; BELLANTI et al., 1966). In a controlled study involving over 1100 subjects, no adverse reactions were seen. Although the outbreak turned out to be due to dengue-3 virus, the incidence of illness in the vaccinated group fell to about one-half or less of that in the control group which had been inoculated with a placebo. The reduction in incidence began 2—3 weeks after vaccination and continued to the end of the epidemic 15 weeks later[1].

A provocative featur of the "MD-1 variant" was the subsequent demonstration that its neurovirulence was somewhat temperature-sensitive in terms of survival of hyperthermic mice and viral yields in their brains (COLE and WISSEMAN, 1969 b). No such temperature dependence was associated with virus that had been subjected to 125 mouse passages and was classified as "highly neurovirulent". The impression seems inescapable that in the "MD-1" derivative temperature sensitivity of neurovirulence was covariant with total loss of human pathogenicity (rash; other signs or symptoms) yet immunogenicity was fully preserved. This fortuitous combination is in accord with findings for other viruses. It is, however, not a predictably reproducible result of intracerebral passages, and brain tissue is not a desirable component of vaccines. Therefore, and in view of the capacity of dengue viruses to replicate in mosquito and in various cell cultures (Section V. A. 3.—4.), it should be preferable to derive ts or otherwise genetically marked avirulent mutants from such sources.

(2) *Are mosquitoes or mosquito cell cultures or vertebrate cell cultures suitable sources of avirulent virus?* The effects of continued passages in mosquitoes (GUBLER and ROSEN, 1976) or mosquito cell cultures (see Section V.) on the pathogenicity of dengue viruses have not been systematically investigated. Models are, however, suggested by the observation that A. *aegypti* or A. *albopictus* cell cultures persistently infected with Sindbis virus (SHENK et al., 1974; STOLLAR et al., 1974; PELEG and STOLLAR, 1974) invariably yield progeny virus that is ts and produces small plaques at permissive temperature. Semliki forest virus from persistently infected A. *aegypti* cell cultures has also been shown to have lower neurovirulence than the mouse-adapted seed virus (PELEG, 1971). Again, similar experiments with dengue viruses are feasible and worthwhile if these features are likely to be associated with lack of human pathogenicity. Any vaccine so derived would have to be extensively purified so as to eliminate sensitization to vector constituents. The stability of the critical mutant character(s) would have to be demonstrated. For Sindbis virus clones from persistently infected A. *albopictus* cells, it has been demonstrated that passage in vertebrate cell cultures, even at 34° C, leads to rapid accumulation of temperature-resistant virus even though it retains the small plaque morphology (SHENK et al., 1974; SCHLESINGER, 1975).

The same safeguards would, of course, be required for virus derived from vertebrate cultures by selection of spontaneous or induced mutants. Here, the scoring of mutant markers (*e.g.*, temperature sensitivity of plaque formation)

---

[1] The observation that dengue-1 vaccine provided partial protection for 3—4 months against type 3 is in tune with SABIN's (1952a) findings in heterotypic challenge experiments (see Section X). It is possible that a cross-protective effect of limited duration may be due to interference rather than conventional immunological phenomena. On the other hand, HALSTEAD et al. (1973a) suggest that the Puerto Rican experiment may be a practical illustration of their findings (see also WHITEHEAD et al., 1970, and discussion in Section XI. A.) that dengue-3 virus, in contrast to the other 3 types, failed consistently to induce viremia in monkeys previously infected with any other type. They reason therefore that it may be possible to eliminate dengue-3 from any vaccination scheme.

would be facilitated, as it has been for other viruses. Again, the basic methodology is at hand, but whether any of the cell lines or strains now known to support dengue virus replication or used for experimental vaccine tests in man (FUJITA *et al.*, 1969) would be acceptable as potential sources for vaccine production is problematic.

(3) *Should vaccines for human use consist of whole virions or immunogenic subunits?* In contrast to the experimental use of attenuated whole virus vaccines (see above), no trials with subunit vaccines have been published. Since it seems likely that the envelope glycoprotein VP-3 is the moiety responsible for, and reacting with, HI and neutralizing antibodies (see Section VI. E.), it would be a logical candidate for such studies. Two questions in need of experimental answers are: (a) does the isolated glycoprotein retain the desired antigenic configuration? (b) does the purification expose new antigenic sites? The latter point is of particular relevance in view of the fact that the antigen involved in immune complex formation in secondary dengue is as yet unidentified (cf. Section X. C.).

A possible alternative approach to vaccine development might be use of the noninfectious SHA fraction which is co-produced with infectious (RHA) virus in cell cultures and mouse brain (see Section VI.). This may offer the advantage of intact antigenic configuration of VP-3 and retention of VP-1 or NV2. On the other hand, SHA has not been obtained completely free of trailing infectious virus.

As with experimental subunit vaccines developed for other kinds of viruses, a key question (other than antigenic integrity and specificity) is whether effective concentrations of antigen(s) can be achieved by methods that are practical for mass production. Another unresolved problem is whether the group B cross-reactive nucleocapsid antigen (VP-2) contributes to the induction of heterospecific immunity.

(4) *Should monovalent or polyvalent or both types of dengue vaccines be developed? Should either type be used in appropriate mixtures or in sequential immunization schemes along with similar preparations of other group B togaviruses?* The hypothetic pros and cons of simultaneous *versus* sequential infections with different dengue serotypes, based mainly on experiments in monkeys, have already been discussed (Section XI. A.). Whether considerations similar to those leading HALSTEAD *et al.* (1973a) to lean in favor of simultaneous immunization would be valid for schemes involving either subunit vaccines or dengue plus other flaviviruses in attenuated forms is an even more speculative issue.

Historically, the notion of the possible effectiveness of mixed or sequential immunization schemes is based not only on the animal models but on a few relevant experiences in volunteer patients. The first deliberate experiments along these lines were reported by SCHLESINGER *et al.* (1956) who vaccinated 17 male adults, of whom eleven received attenuated dengue-2 virus alone (suckling mouse brain, New Guinea B strain), three dengue-2 plus yellow fever 17D vaccine, and three dengue-1 (suckling mouse brain, Hawaii strain) plus dengue-2 plus 17D vaccine. With the mixtures inoculated subcutaneously, dengue-2 appeared to be the dominant immunogen, in the sense that post-vaccination neutralization indices against the other two viruses were relatively low. A byproduct of these early tests was the *post hoc* revelation that four volunteers, who gave an unexpectedly strong and rapid antibody response reactive with all three viruses (3 had received only monovalent dengue-2 vaccine), had been vaccinated against yellow fever

7—8 years previously—a fact they had not revealed to the experimenters. Challenge experiments were unsuccessful due to inactivation of the viruses used.

Various mixtures or sequences of attenuated dengue-1 (Mochizuki strain) and 17 D YF vaccines were given by Fujita *et al.* (1969). They too observed a suggestion of one-way interference with antibody production. On the other hand, they found no evidence for a "booster" effect on dengue-1 or YF antibody production in individuals who may have had prior exposure to JE virus. Challenge inoculations were not reported.

It is of interest to reiterate that Wisseman *et al.* (1966) found that volunteers who had a history of inapparent infection with JE virus followed by YF vaccination and whose serum contained antibodies neutralizing dengue-1 virus were not protected against experimental dengue-1 infection but developed the full-blown clinical disease. This result suggests, as indicated before, that something other than mere presence of cross-reactive antibody is required for effective clinical immunity.

(5) *What are some considerations that might encourage or discourage the use of one or another type of vaccine?* It is clear from the foregoing discussion that, even judging from the meagre experience with the use of experimental vaccines in man, (a) the methodology for constructing vaccines is available, (b) effective homotypic protection can be induced by attenuated virus vaccines. A central question is, however, whether and under what conditions the use of active immunization procedures is desirable or indicated. The antigenic complexity and subgroup-specific heterogeneity of dengue viruses, combined with their mandatory mosquito—man—mosquito—man ... transmission cycle, creates nosological-epidemiological problems quite without parallels among other human virus diseases.

(a) Classical primary dengue is, as a rule, a non-fatal disease. Even considering the exceptions to this generalization, noted in Section X, the fatality rate and incidence of sequelae is probably lower than for any other virus disease for which large-scale vaccination has ever been considered. Clinical manifestations of primary infection in young children in highly endemic areas are reported to be extremely mild (Halstead *et al.*, 1969a) or absent (Ventura *et al.*, 1975). These circumstances magnify in a unique way the dilemma of weighing the risks inherent in vaccination against the infinitesimally small danger associated with primary dengue: the vaccine must be "absolutely safe"—perhaps safer than any vaccines in current use. Special contingencies such as possible military emergency needs are not considered here.

(b) The occurrence of dengue epidemics in territories where it has not been prevalent before indicates the existence of an epidemiological setting (introduction of virus, vector density, density of susceptible human population) favoring endemic establishment *plus* simultaneous or subsequent superimposition of additional serotypes: according to the "second-infection" hypothesis, this may set the stage for the appearance of DHF and DSS. The events of recent years in the Caribbean (dengue-3 in 1963, dengue-2 and -3 in 1968—1969) serve as an example in which the latter complications have *not yet* been observed. However, as pointed out by Ehrenkranz *et al.* (1971) for this situation, ". . . The implications of continuing dengue epidemics in Caribbean countries are not trivial for themselves or their neighbors. For the community, a dengue epidemic can be an economic disaster. The loss of an effective work force for several days, followed by their inefficient function for several weeks thereafter, is no small matter. Moreover, the associated publicity frequently discourages travel to these areas and damages the economy, which is generally dependent on tourism. The recent increase in tempo of epidemics in the Carribean raises the possibility of the occurrence of urban hyperendemicity of dengue without major epidemics. This took place in tropical Asia between 1902 and 1950, and seems to have been a prelude to the catastrophic epidemics of dengue shock syndrome that began in 1953. In some endemic areas in Asia, human infections with all four dengue types are observed with a sixmonth period. The presence of both dengue viruses 2 and 3 in the Caribbean 1968—1969 epidemic may be a portent of these more serious developments ... Vaccine development poses some unusual theoretical problems. A vaccine virus that induces only homotypic protection could itself sensitize and set the stage for the dengue shock syndrome, if infection with different serotypes subsequently occurred ... The increasing size of human population in the Caribbean, the continued presence of *A. aegypti*, the lack of lasting heterotypic protection and the absence of knowledge of origin of epidemics all point to continuing difficulties with dengue.''

(c) These considerations bring us to the shock syndrome as a sufficiently serious and life-threatening condition perhaps to warrant modification of the stringent ''no risk'' requirements postulated under (a) above. Its limitation to young children in those countries in which it has been endemic (Section X. C.) imposes further stringencies: (i) none of the vaccines thus far used experimentally have been tested in children of the critical age group; (ii) there remain unanswered questions regarding possible age-specific physiological factors which may account for the immunopathological response, and these may alter the response to vaccination — especially sequential schemes—as well.

XII. Opportunities for the Future

This monograph ends with a lengthy and rather inconclusive discussion on the current status of dengue vaccines for use of man. This emphasis is deliberate: the practical solution of pressing medical problems through prophylaxis or therapy is, after all, an ultimate aim of ''basic'' and ''applied'' research on infectious diseases; the inconclusiveness shows how much more needs to be learned.

Among all known viruses causing human disease, the dengue viruses as a group are unique. They form a distinctive subgroup—four known antigenic types—of a larger genus, the group B togaviruses or flaviviruses, with which they share structural properties and at least one common antigen. What makes them genetically, biochemically, biologically, and immunologically distinct from the other members? There is no other group of four closely related, yet immunologically distinguishable, viruses of which one can so sensitize a human being that reinfection with another may cause a lifethreatening shock reaction. What are the specific determinants shared or not shared by the four dengue serotypes? What is the nature of the antigen(s) and antibodies responsible for immune complex formation in second heterotypic infections? What is the pathogenesis of the immunological lesions leading to hemorrhagic fever or shock? Are there physiological functions other than immunological that restrict the occurrence of endemic DHF and DSS to young children? Why have these complications arisen in endemic proportions in Southern and Southeast Asia but not in other regions harboring more than one type of dengue virus? Does the mandatory mosquito—man—mosquito—man ... transmission cycle impose on these viruses special selective pressures that have not expressed themselves similarly in other closely related arboviruses?

These and other open questions raised throughout this treatise make for one of the most fascinating challenges for virologists, molecular biologists, immunologists, as well as for clinicians and epidemiologists. Progress during the last three decades has been impressive mainly by exposing these challenges and by setting the stage, technically and conceptually, for meeting them.

Acknowledgments

I am grateful to my associates, past and present, who have kept dengue research going in our laboratory, especially Drs. Jack W. Frankel, Joseph W. Winter, Thomas M. Stevens, Irene T. Schulze, Takeo Matsumura, and Victor Stollar. Our work has been supported by the United States-Japan Cooperative Medical Science Program through Public Health Service Grant No. AI-05920 (formerly E 113 and AI-01129).

Thanks are due Colonel Phillip K. Russell and Dr. Scott B. Halstead for sharing with me manuscripts and stimulating discussions.

Mrs. Frances Huttemann has earned my gratitude for heroically and uncomplainingly typing unending versions of the manuscript, thus bringing order out of chaos.

References

ADA, G. L., ANDERSON, S. G.: The infectivity of preparations made by the action of phenol on dengue I, dengue II, GD VII and Herpes simplex viruses. Aust. J. biol. Sci. **21**, 159 (1959).

AGRAWAL, H. O., BRUENING, G.: Isolation of high molecular weight P^{32}-labeled influenza virus ribonucleic acid. Proc. nat. Acad. Sci. (Wash.) **55**, 818—825 (1966).

AOKI, H., EYLAR, O. R., WISSEMAN, C. L., JR.: A plaque assay of dengue viruses in BHK-21 cell cultures and *in vitro* studies. Annual Reports from the Department of Microbiology, University of Maryland School of Medicine (1967).

ASHBURN, P. M., CRAIG, C. F.: Experimental investigations regarding the etiology of dengue fever. J. infect. Dis. **4**, 440—475 (1907).

ATCHISON, R. W., ORDONEZ, J. V., SATHER, G. E., HAMMON, W. McD.: Fluorescent antibody, complement fixation method for detection of dengue viruses in mice. J. Immunol. **96**, 936—943 (1966).

BALTIMORE, D.: Expression of animal virus genomes. Bact. Rev. **35**, 235—241 (1971).

BANCROFT, T. L.: On the aetiology of dengue fever. Aust. med. Gaz. **25**, 17—18 (1906).

BANERJEE, K.: Evaluation of the effect of fresh serum factor in the neutralization of dengue viruses. Indian J. med. Res. **55**, 405—410 (1967).

BANERJEE, K.: Observations on certain biological markers of dengue viruses (with a note on the relationship between virus dose and survival time in mice). Indian J. med. Res. **57**, 1165—1180 (1969a).

BANERJEE, K.: Observations on certain parameters for the growth and assay of dengue viruses in tissue culture. Indian J. med. Res. **58**, 30—38 (1969b).

BANERJEE, K., SINGH, K. R. P.: Establishment of carrier cultures of *Aedes albopictus* cell line infected with arboviruses. Indian J. med. Res. **56**, 812—814 (1968).

BANTA, J. E.: Cultivation of dengue, Western equine encephalitis, Japanese B encephalitis, and West Nile viruses in selected mammalian cell cultures. Amer. J. Hyg. **67**, 286—299 (1958)

BARNES, W. J. S., ROSEN, L.: Fatal hemorrhagic disease and shock associated with primary dengue infection on a Pacific island. Amer. J. trop. Med. Hyg. **23**, 495—506 (1974).

BEASLEY, A. R., LICHTER, W., SIGEL, M. M.: Studies on latent infections of tissue cultures with dengue virus. Arch. ges. Virusforsch. **10**, 672—683 (1960).

BELLANTI, J.A., BOURKE, R. T. C., BUESCHER, E. L., CADIGAN, F. C., COLE, G. A., ELBATAWI, Y., WATGI, J. N., McCOWN, J. M., NEGRON, H., ORDONEZ, J. V., SCHEIDER, F. G., SMITH, T., WARRAM, J. M., WISSEMAN, C. L., JR.: Report of dengue vaccine field trial in the Caribbean, 1963: A collaborative study. Bull. Wld Hlth Org. **35**, 93 (1966).

BERGE, T. O.: International Catalogue of Arboviruses, 2nd Edition. U.S. Dept. of HEW Publ. No. (CDC) 75—8301, 789 pp. (1975).

BERGOLD, G. H., MAZZALI, R.: Plaque formation by arboviruses. J. gen. Virol. **2**, 273—284 (1968).

BHAMARAPRAVATI, N., HALSTEAD, S. B., SOOKAVACHANA, PL., BOONYAPAKNAVIK, V.: Studies on dengue virus infection. I. Immunofluorescent localization of virus in mouse tissue. Arch. Path. **77**, 538—543 (1964).

BHAMARAPRAVATI, N., TOOCHINDA, P., BOONYAPAKNAVIK, V.: Pathology of Thailand haemorrhagic fever: A study of 100 autopsy cases. Amer. J. trop. Med. Parasit. **61**, 500—510 (1967).

BLANC, G., CAMINOPETROS, J.: Recherches expérimentales sur la dengue. Ann. Inst. Pasteur **44**, 367—436 (1930).

BLANC, G., CAMINOPETROS, J., DUMAS, J., SAENZ, A.: Recherches expérimentales sur la sensibilité des singes inférieurs au virus de la dengue. C. R. Acad. Sci. (Paris) **188**, 468—470 (1929).

BLANC, G., CAMINOPETROS, J., MANOUSSAKIS, E.: Quelques recherches expérimentales sur la dengue. Bull. Soc. Path. exot. **21**, 525—537 (1928).

BOKISCH, V. A., TOP, F. H., JR., RUSSELL, P. K., DIXON, F. J., MÜLLER-EBERHARD, H. J.: The potential pathogenic role of complement in dengue hemorrhagic shock syndrome. New Engl. J. Med. **289**, 996—1000 (1973).

BOND, J. O., HAMMON, W. McD.: Epidemiologic studies of possible cross protection between dengue and St. Louis encephalitis arboviruses in Florida. Amer. J. Epidem. **92**, 321—329 (1970).

BOULTON, R. W., WESTAWAY, E. G.: Comparisons of togaviruses: Sindbis virus (group A) and Kunjin virus (group B). Virology **49**, 283—289 (1972).

BOULTON, R. W., WESTAWAY, E. G.: Replication of the flavivirus Kunjin: proteins, glycoproteins, and maturation associated with cell membranes. Virology **69**, 416 to 430 (1976).

BRANDT, W. E., BUESCHER, E. L., HETRICK, F. M.: Production and characterization of arbovirus antibody in mouse ascitic fluid. Amer. J. trop. Med. Hyg. **16**, 339—347 (1967).

BRANDT, W. E., CARDIFF, R. D., RUSSELL, P. K.: Dengue virions and antigens in brain and serum of infected mice. J. Virol. **6**, 500—506 (1970).

BRANDT, W. E., RUSSELL, P. K.: Influence of cell type and virus upon virus-specific immune cytolysis. Infect. & Immun. **11**, 330—333 (1974).

BRANDT, W. E., SMITH, T. J., BUESCHER, E. L., RUSSELL, P. K.: Purification and characteristics of a dengue virus, complement-fixing, soluble antigen. Bact. Proc., p. 186 (1969) (Abstract).

BRAWNER, T. A., LEE, J. C., TRENT, D. W.: Nuclear and cytoplasmic localization of polyadenylate rich St. Louis encephalitis (SLE) virus induced RNA. Abstracts of Ann. Mtg. Amer. Soc. Microbiol., p. 202 (1973).

BUCKLEY, S. M.: Serial propagation of types 1, 2, 3, and 4 dengue virus in HeLa cells with concomitant cytopathic effect. Nature (Lond.) **192**, 778—779 (1961).

BUCKLEY, S. M., SRIHONGSE, S.: Production of hemagglutinin by dengue virus in HeLa cells. Proc. Soc. exp. Biol. (N.Y.) **113**, 284—288 (1963).

CARDIFF, R. D., BRANDT, W. E., McCLOUD, T. G., SHAPIRO, D.. RUSSELL, P. K.: Immunological and biophysical separation of dengue-2 antigens. J. Virol. **7**, 15—23 (1971).

CARDIFF, R. D., McCLOUD, T. G., BRANDT, W. E., RUSSELL, P. K.: Molecular size and charge relationships of the soluble complement-fixing antigens of dengue viruses. Virology **41**, 569—572 (1970).

CARDIFF, R. D., RUSS, S. B., BRANDT, W. E., RUSSELL, P. K.: RNA polymerase in group B arbovirus (dengue-2) infected cells. Arch. ges. Virusforsch. **40**, 392—396 (1973a).

CARDIFF, R. D., RUSS, S. B., BRANDT, W. E., RUSSELL, P. K.: Cytological localization of dengue-2 antigens: An immunological study with ultrastructural correlation. Infect. & Immun. **7**, 809—816 (1973b).

CAREY, D. E.: Chikungunya and Dengue: A case of mistaken identity? J. Hist. Med. **26**, 243—262 (1971).

CAREY, D. E., MYERS, R. M., REUBEN, R.: Dengue types 1 and 4 viruses in wild-caught mosquitoes in South India. Science **143**, 131—132 (1964).

CAREY, D. E., MYERS, R. M., RODRIGUES, F. M.: Two episodes of dengue fever, caused by types 4 and 1 viruses, in an individual previously immunized against yellow fever. Amer. J. trop. Med. Hyg. **14**, 448—450 (1965).

CASALS, J.: Problems encountered in the classification and nomenclature of the arthropod-borne viruses (Arboviruses). Amer. J. Epidem. **88**, 147—148 (1968a).

CASALS, J.: Filtration of arboviruses through "Millipore" membranes. Nature (Lond.) **217**, 648—649 (1968b).

CASALS, J., BROWN, L. V.: Hemagglutination with arthropod-borne viruses. J. exp. Med. **99**, 429—449 (1954).

CATANZARO, P. J., BRANDT, E. W., HOGREFE, W. R., RUSSELL, P. K.: Detection of dengue cell-surface antigens by peroxidase-labeled antibodies and immune cytolysis. Infect & Immun. **10**, 381—388 (1974).

CATANZARO, P. J., BRANDT, W. E., RUSSELL, P. K.: The influence of arboviral infection on the susceptibility of cultured cells to immune injury *in vitro*. Amer. J. Path. **80**, 91—100 (1975).

CHAN, Y. C.: Rapid typing of dengue viruses by micro-precipitin agar-gel diffusion technique. Nature (Lond.) **206**, 116—117 (1965).

CHAPPELL, W. A., CALISHER, C. H., TOOLE, R. A., MANESS, K. C., SASSO, D. R., HENDERSON, B. E.: Comparison of three methods listed to isolate dengue virus type 2. Appl. Microbiol. **22**, 1100—1103 (1971).

CLARKE, D. H.: Antigenic analysis of certain group B arthropod-borne viruses by antibody absorption. J. exp. Med. **111**, 1—20 (1960).

CLARKE, D. H., CASALS, J.: Techniques for hemagglutination and hemagglutination-inhibition with arthropod-borne viruses. Amer. J. trop. Med. Hyg. **7**, 561—573 (1958).

CLELAND, J. B., BRADLEY, B., McDONALD, W.: On the transmission of Australian dengue by the mosquito *Stegomyia fasciata*. Med. J. Aust. **2**, 179—200 (1916).

CLELAND, J. B., BRADLEY, B., McDONALD, W.: Further experiments in the aetiology of dengue fever. J. Hyg. (Lond.) **18**, 217—254 (1919).

COLE, G. A., WISSEMAN, C. L., JR.: Pathogenesis of type 1 dengue virus infection in suckling, weanling and adult mice. I. The relation of virus replication to interferon and antibody formation. Amer. J. Epidem. **89**, 669—680 (1969a).

COLE, G. A., WISSEMAN, C. L., JR.: The effect of hyperthermia on dengue virus infection of mice. Proc. Soc. exp. Biol. (N.Y.) **130**, 359—363 (1969b).

COLEMAN, J. C., McLEAN, D. M.: Dengue virus transmission by *Aedes aegypti* mosquitoes following intrathoracic inoculation. Amer. J. trop. Med. Hyg. **22**, 124—129 (1973).

COPANARIS, P.: L'épidemie de dengue en Grèce au cours de l'été 1928. Bull. Off. int. Hyg. publ. **20**, 1590—1601 (1928).

CORY, J., YUNKER, C. E.: Arbovirus plaques in mosquito cell monolayers. Acta virol. **16**, 90 (1972).

CRAIG, C. F.: On the nature of the virus of yellow fever, dengue, and Pappataci fever. N.Y. med. J. **93**, 360—369 (1911).

CRAIG, C. F.: The etiology of dengue fever. J. Amer. med. Ass. **75**, 1171—1176 (1920).

CRAIGHEAD, J. E., SATHER, G. E., HAMMON, W. McD., DAMMIN, G. J.: Pathology of dengue virus infections in mice. Arch. Path. **81**, 232—239 (1966).

CUADRADO, R. R., CASALS, J.: Differentiation of arboviruses by immunoelectrophoresis. J. Immunol. **98**, 314—320 (1967).

DALRYMPLE, J. M., VOGEL, S. N., TERAMOTO, A. Y., RUSSELL, P. K.: Antigenic components of group A arboviruses. J. Virol. **12**, 1034—1042 (1973).

DEFENDI, V., LEHMAN, J., KRAEMER, P.: "Morphologically normal" hamster cells with malignant properties. Virology **19**, 592—598 (1963).

DELLER, J. J., JR., RUSSELL, P. K.: An analysis of fevers of unknown origin in American soldiers in Vietnam. Ann. int. Med. **66**, 1129—1143 (1967).

DEMADRID, A. T., PORTERFIELD, J. S.: A simple micro-culture method for the study of group B arboviruses. Bull. Wld Hlth Org. **40**, 113—121 (1969).

DEMADRID, A. T., PORTERFIELD, J. S.: The flaviviruses (group B arboviruses): A cross-neutralization study. J. gen. Virol. **23**, 91—96 (1974).

DEMSEY, A., STEERE, R. L., BRANDT, W. E., VELTRI, B. J.: Morphology and development of dengue-2 virus employing the freeze-fracture and thin-section techniques. J. Ultrastruct. Res. **46**, 102—116 (1974).

DIERCKS, F. H.: Isolation of a type 2 dengue virus by use of hamster kidney cell cultures. Amer. J. trop. Med. Hyg. **8**, 488—491 (1959).

DIERCKS, F. H., HAMMON, W. McD.: Hamster kidney cell tissue cultures for propagation of Japanese B encephalitis virus. Proc. Soc. exp. Biol. (N.Y.) **97**, 627—632 (1958).

DONALD, H. B., ISAACS, A.: Counts of influenza virus particles. J. gen. Microbiol. **10**, 457—464 (1954).

EAGLE, H.: Nutritional needs of mammalian cells in tissue culture. Science **122**, 501—504 (1955).

EDELMAN, R., NISALAK, A., PARIYANONDA, A., ODOMSAKDI, S., JOHNSEN, D. O.: Immunoglobulin response and viremia in dengue-vaccinated gibbons repeatedly challenged with Japanese encephalitis virus. Amer. J. Epidem. **97**, 208—218 (1973).

EDELMAN, R., PARIYANONDA, A.: Human immunoglobulin M antibody in the serodiagnosis of Japanese encephalitis virus infections. Amer. J. Epidem. **98**, 29—38 (1973).

EHRENKRANZ, N. J., VENTURA, A. K., CUADRADO, P. R., POND, W. L., PORTER, J. E.: Pandemic dengue in Caribbean countries and the Southern United States—past, present and potential problems. New Engl. J. Med. **285**, 1460—1469 (1971).

FALKLER, W. A., JR., DIWAN, A. R., HALSTEAD, S. B.: Human antibody to dengue soluble complement-fixing (SCF) antigens. J. Immunol. **111**, 1804—1809 (1973).

FAZEKAS DE ST. GROTH, S.: The neutralization of viruses. Advanc. Virus Res. **9**, 1—125 (1962).

FENNER, F.: Classification and nomenclature of viruses: the current position. ASM News (Amer. Soc. for Microbiol.) **42**, 170—173 (1976).

FINDLAY, G. M.: The relation between dengue and Rift Valley fever. Trans. roy. Soc. trop. Med. Hyg. **26**, 157—160 (1932).

FISCHER, D. B., HALSTEAD, S. B.: Observations related to pathogenesis of dengue hemorrhagic fever. V. Examination of age specific sequential infection rates using a mathematical model. Yale J. Biol. Med. **42**, 329—349 (1970).

FRAENKEL-CONRAT, H.: The small RNA viruses of plants, animals and bacteria. B. Chemical properties. In: Molecular Basis of Virology, ACS Monograph (FRAENKEL-CONRAT, H., ed.), pp. 134—168. New York-Amsterdam-London: Reinhold Book Corp. 1968.

FUJITA, N., ODA, K., YASUI, Y., HOTTA, S.: Research on dengue in tissue culture. IV. Serologic responses of human beings to combined inoculations of attenuated, tissue-cultured type 1 dengue virus and yellow fever vaccine. Kobe J. med. Sci. **15**. 163 to 180 (1969).

FUJITA, N., TAMURA, M., HOTTA, S.: Dengue virus plaque formation on microplate cultures and its application to virus neutralization. Proc. Soc. exp. Biol. (N.Y.) **148**. 472—475 (1975).

GAROFF, H., SIMONS, K., RENKONEN, O.: Isolation and characterization of the membrane proteins of Semliki Forest virus. Virology **61**, 493—504 (1974).

GEORGIADES, J., STIM, T. B., McCOLLUM, R. W., HENDERSON, J. R.: Dengue virus plaque formation in rhesus monkey kidney cultures. Proc. Soc. exp. Biol. (N.Y.) **118**, 385—388 (1965).

GIBBS, A. J., HARRISON, B. D.: Realistic approach to virus classification and nomenclature. Nature (Lond.) **218**, 927—929 (1968).

GIBBS, A. J., HARRISON, B. D.. WATSON, D. H., WILDY, O.: What's in a virus name? Nature (Lond.) **209**, 450 (1966).

GORMAN, B., GOSS, P.: Sensitivity of arboviruses to proteases. J. gen. Virol. **16**, 83—86 (1972).

GRAHAM, H.: The dengue: A study of its pathology and mode of propagation. J. trop. Med. **6**, 209—214 (1903).

GRIFFITHS, B. B., GRANT, L. S., MINOTT, O. D., BELLE, E. A.: An epidemic of dengue-like illness in Jamaica—1963. Amer. J. trop. Med. Hyg. **17**, 584—589 (1968).

GROSSBERG, S. E., SCHERER, W. F.: Immunity in group B arthropod-borne virus diseases. Accidental dengue I virus infection in a laboratory worker with antibodies to Japanese encephalitis virus. Amer. J. Hyg. **69**, 60—67 (1958).

GROSSMAN, R. A., EDELMAN, R., CHIEWANICH, P., VOODHIKUL, P., SIRIWAN, C.: Study of Japanese encephalitis virus in Chiangmai Valley, Thailand. II. Human clinical infections. Amer. J. Epidem. **98**, 121—132 (1973a).

GROSSMAN, R. A., EDELMAN, R., WILLHIGHT, M., PANTUWATANA, S., UDOMSAKDI, S.: Study of Japanese encephalitis virus in Chiangmai Valley, Thailand. III. Human seroepidemiology and inapparent infection. Amer. J. Epidem. **98**, 133—149 (1973b).

GROSSMAN, R. A., EDELMAN, R., GOULD, D. J.: Study of Japanese encephalitis virus in Chiangmai Valley, Thailand. VI. Summary and conclusions. Amer. J. Epidem. **100**, 69—76 (1974).

GROSSMAN, R. A., GOULD, D. J., SMITH, T. J., JOHNSEN, D. O., PANTUWATANA, S.: Study of Japanese encephalitis virus in Chiangmai Valley, Thailand. I. Introduction and study design. Amer. J. Epidem. **98**, 111—120 (1973c).

GUBLER, D. J., ROSEN, L.: A simple technique for demonstrating transmission of dengue virus by mosquitoes without the use of vertebrate hosts. Amer. J. trop. Med. Hyg. **25**, 146—150 (1976).

HALLAUER, C., KRONAUER, G.: Nachweis von Gelbfiebervirus-Haemagglutinin in menschlichen Explantaten. Arch. ges. Virusforsch. **10**, 267—286 (1960).

HALSTEAD, S. B.: Dengue and hemorrhagic fevers of Southeast Asia: With discussion by Max Theiler. Yale J. Biol. Med. **37**, 434—454 (1965).

HALSTEAD, S. B.: Mosquito-borne hemorrhagic fevers of South and South-East Asia. Bull. Wld Hlth Org. **35**, 3—15 (1966).

HALSTEAD, S. B.: Observations related to pathogenesis of dengue hemorrhagic fever. VI. Hypotheses and discussion. Yale J. Biol. Med. **42**, 350—362 (1970).

HALSTEAD, S. B.: Epidemiological aspects of dengue and chikungunya infections. I. Conventional disease manifestations. Proc. of Conference on the Pathogenesis of Arboviral Infections, Vol. I, 33—67. U.S.-Japan Coop. Med. Sci. Program, Panels on Viral Diseases, Honolulu, Hawaii, September, 1971.

HALSTEAD, S. B.: Etiologies of the experimental dengues of Siler and Simmons. Amer. J. trop. Med. Hyg. **23**, 974—982 (1974).

HALSTEAD, S. B., CASALS, J., SHOTWELL, H., PALUMBO, N.: Studies on the immunization of monkeys against dengue. I. Protection derived from single and sequential virus infection. Amer. J. trop. Med. Hyg. **22**, 365—374 (1973a).

HALSTEAD, S. B., CHOW, J. S., MARCHETTE, N. J.: Immunological enhancement of dengue virus replication. Nature (N.B.) **243**, 24—25 (1973b).

HALSTEAD, S. B., NIMMANNITYA, S., COHEN, S. N.: Observations related to pathogenesis of dengue hemorrhagic fever. IV. Relation of disease severity to antibody response and virus recovered. Yale J. Biol. Med. **42**, 311—328 (1970c).

HALSTEAD, S. B., NIMMANNITAY, S., MARGIOTTA, M. R.: Dengue and chikungunya virus infection in man in Thailand, 1962—1964. II. Observations on disease in outpatients. Amer. J. trop. Med. Hyg. **18**, 972—983 (1969a).

HALSTEAD, S. B., NIMMANNITYA, S., YAMARAT, C., RUSSELL, P. K.: Hemorrhagic fever in Thailand newer knowledge regarding etiology. Jap. J. med. Sci. Biol. **20**, 96—103 (1967).

HALSTEAD, S. B., PALUMBO, N.: Studies on the immunization of monkeys against dengue. II. Protection following inoculation of combinations of viruses. Amer. J. trop. Med. Hyg. **22**, 375—381 (1973).

HALSTEAD, S. B., SCANLON, J. E., UMPAIVIT, P., UDOMSADKI, S.: Dengue and chikungunya virus infection in man in Thailand, 1962—1964. IV. Epidemiologic studies in the Bangkok metropolitan area. Amer. J. trop. Med. Hyg. **18**, 997—1021 (1969c).

HALSTEAD, S. B., SHOTWELL, H., CASALS, J.: Studies on the pathogenesis of dengue infection in monkeys. I. Clinical laboratory responses to primary infection. J. infect. Dis. **128**, 7—14 (1973c).

HALSTEAD, S. B., SHOTWELL, H., CASALS, J.: Studies on the pathogenesis of dengue infection in monkeys. II. Clinical laboratory responses to heterologous infection. J. infect. Dis. **128**, 15—22 (1973d).

HALSTEAD, S. B., SUKHAVACHANA, P., NISALAK, A.: *In vitro* recovery of dengue viruses from naturally infected human beings and arthropods. Nature (Lond.) **202**, 931—932 (1964a).

HALSTEAD, S. B., SIKHAVACHANA, P., NISALAK, A.: Assay of mouse-adapted dengue viruses in mammalian cell cultures by an interference method. Proc. Soc. exp. Biol. (N.Y.) **115**, 1062—1068 (1964b).

HALSTEAD, S. B., UDONSAKDI, S., SCANLON, J. E., ROHITAYODHIN, S.: Dengue and chikungunya virus infection in man in Thailand, 1962—1964. V. Epidemiologic observations outside Bangkok. Amer. J. trop. Med. Hyg. **18**, 1022—1033 (1969d).

HALSTEAD, S. B., SIMASTHIEN, P.: Observations related to pathogenesis of dengue hemorrhagic fever. II. Antigenic and biologic properties of dengue viruses and their association with disease response in the host. Yale J. Biol. Med. **42**, 276—292 (1970b).

HALSTEAD, S. B., UDOMSAKDI, S., SIMASTHIEN, P., SINGHARAJ, P., SIKHAVACHANA, P., NISALAK, A.: Observations related to pathogenesis of dengue hemorrhagic fever. I. Experience with clarification of dengue viruses. Yale J. Biol. Med. **42**, 261—275 (1970a).

HALSTEAD, S. B., UDOMSAKDI, S., SINGHARAJ, P., NISALAK, A.: Dengue and chikungunya virus infection in man in Thailand, 1962—1964. III. Clinical, epidemiologic, and virologic observations on disease in non-indigenous white persons. Amer. J. trop. Med. Hyg. **18**, 984—986 (1969b).

HAMMON, W. McD.: Dengue and dengue-related diseases. In: Cecil-Loeb Textbook of Medicine, 11th ed., pp. 92—97. Philadelphia-London: W. B. Saunders Co. 1963.

HAMMON, W. McD.: Observations on dengue fever, benign protector and killer: A Dr. Jekyll and Mr. Hyde. Amer. J. trop. Med. Hyg. **18**, 159—165 (1969).

HAMMON, W. McD.: Dengue hemorrhagic fever—Do we know its cause? Amer. J. trop. Med. Hyg. **22**, 82—91 (1973).

HAMMON, W. McD., RUDNICK, A., SATHER, G. E.: Viruses associated with hemorrhagic fevers of the Philippines and Thailand. Science **131**, 1102—1103 (1960a).

HAMMON, W. McD., RUDNICK, A., SATHER, G., ROGERS, K. D.: The etiology of Philippine hemorrhagic fever and its relation to dengue, from Proc. 6th Int. Congr. on trop. Med. and Malaria, Vol. V, pp. 107—111 (1958).

HAMMON, W. McD., RUDNICK, A., SATHER, G.E., ROGERS, K. D., CHAN, V., DIZON, J. J., BASACA-SEVILLA, V.: Studies on Philippine hemorrhagic fever: Relationship

to dengue viruses. Proc. 9th Pacific Sci. Congr. Bangkok. Thailand, pp. 67—72
(1957).

HAMMON, W. McD., RUDNICK, A., SATHER, G., ROGERS, K. D., MORSE, L. J.: New
hemorrhagic fevers of children in the Philippines and Thailand. Trans. Ass. Amer.
Phycns 73, 140—155 (1960b).

HAMMON, W. McD., SATHER, G. E.: Virological findings in the 1960 hemorrhagic fever
epidemic (dengue) in Thailand. Amer. J. trop. Med. Hyg. 13, 629—641 (1964a).

HAMMON, W. McD., SATHER, G. E.: Problems of typing dengue viruses. Milit. Med.
129, 130—135 (1964b).

HAMMON, W. McD., SATHER, G. E., BOND, J. O., LEWIS, F. Y.: Effect of previous
dengue infection and yellow fever vaccination on St. Louis encephalitis virus
serological surveys in Tampa Bay area of Florida. Amer. J. Epidem. 83, 571—585
(1966).

HAMMON, W. McD., SATHER, G. E., RUDNICK, A.: Identification and classification of
the dengue group of viruses. Proc. Symp. Thai Haemorrhagic Fever, SEATO Med.
Res. Monograph, No. 2, pp. 30—36 (1961a).

HANNOUN, C., ECHALIER, G.: Arbovirus multiplication in an established diploid cell
line of *Drosophila melanogaster*. Curr. Top. Microbiol. Immunol. 55, 227—230
(1971).

HASHIMOTO, K.: Fundamental studies on the purification of dengue virus. I. Studies
on the stabilities for the physical and chemical influences. Kurume Igakkai Zasshi
(J. Kurume Med. Assoc.) 17, 384—394 (1954).

HASHIMOTO, K.: Studies on the fundamental character of dengue virus. II. Studies on
the partial purification by use of the stabilities for various chemical agents. Kurume
Igakkai Zasshi (J. Kurume Med. Assoc.) 18, 152—161 (1955).

HATGI, J. N., WISSEMAN, C. L., JR., ROSENZWEIG, E. C., HARRINGTON, B. R., KITAOKA,
M.: Immunological studies with group B arthropod-borne viruses. VI. Hemagglu-
tination-inhibiting antibody responses to 17D yellow fever vaccine in human subjects with different degress of complexitity of prevaccination group B virus experience. Amer. J. trop. Med. Hyg. 15, 601—610 (1966).

HAWKES, R. A., MARSHALL, I. D.: Studies of arboviruses by agar gel diffusion. Amer.
J. Epidem. 86, 28—44 (1967).

HELLER, E.: Enhancement of chikungunya virus replication and inhibition of interferon production by actinomycin D. Virology 21, 652—656 (1963).

HENLE, W., HENLE, G., DEINHARDT, R., BERGS, V.: Studies on persistent infections
of tissue cultures. J. exp. Med. 110, 525—541 (1959).

HIROKI, H., AKISADA, T., OKADA, Y., KURASHIMA, Y.: Studies on dengue. I. Inoculation of dengue virus into the ground squirrel (*Citellus mongolicus ramosus* Thomas).
Proc. 18th Ann. Mtg., Jap. Bact. Soc., pp. 62—63 (1944).

HOFFMAN, J. M., MERTENS, W. K., SNIJDERS, E. P.: The transport of the Javanese
"endemic dengue" to Amsterdam. Proc. Acad. Sci. Amsterdam 32, 909—910 (1932).

HOLMES, I. H., WARBURTON, M. F.: Is rubella an arbovirus? Lancet ii, 1233—1236
(1967).

HOLMES, I. H., WARK, M. C., WARBURTON, M. F.: Is rubella an arbovirus? II. Ultrastructural morphology and development. Virology 37, 15—25 (1969).

HORZINEK, M. C.: Comparative aspects of togaviruses. J. gen. Virol. 20, 87—103
(1973a).

HORZINEK, M. C.: The Structure of togaviruses. Progr. med. Virol. 16, 109—156
(1973b).

HOTTA, S.: Histopathology of dengue infection in mice. Tokyo Iji Shinshi (Tokyo
Med. J.) 68, 19—23 (1951).

HOTTA, S.: Experimental studies on dengue. I. Isolation, identification and modification of the virus. J. infect. Dis. 90, 1—19 (1952).

HOTTA, S.: Partial purification of the mouse-adapted dengue virus. Acta Schol. med.
Univ. Kioto 31, 7—10 (1953).

HOTTA, S.: Experiments of active immunization against dengue with mouse-passaged
unmodified virus. Acta trop. (Basel) 11, 97—104 (1954).

HOTTA, S.: Twenty years of laboratory experience with dengue virus. In: Applied Virology (SANDERS, M., LENNETTE, E. H., eds.), pp. 228—256. Wisconsin: Olympic Press 1965.

HOTTA, S.: Dengue and Related Hemorrhagic Diseases. St. Louis, Green, Inc., publishers, 166 pp. (1969).

HOTTA, S., EVANS, C. A.: Cultivation of mouse-adapted dengue virus (type 1) in rhesus monkey tissue culture. J. infect. Dis. 98, 88—97 (1956a).

HOTTA, S., EVANS, C. A.: Cultivation of type 2 dengue virus in rhesus kidney tissue culture. Proc. Soc. exp. Biol. (N.Y.) 93, 153—155 (1956b).

HOTTA, S., EVANS, C. A.: Ether-sensitivity of dengue virus. Virology 2, 704—706 (1956c).

HOTTA, S., FUJITA, N., MARUYAMA, T.: Research on dengue in tissue culture. I. Plaque formation in an established monkey kidney cell line culture. Kobe J. med. Sci. 12, 179—187 (1966a).

HOTTA, S., OHYAMA, A., YAMADA, T., AWAI, T.: Cultivation of mouse-passaged dengue viruses in human and animal tissue cultures. Jap. J. Microbiol. 5, 77—88 (1961).

HOTTA, S., SHIOMI, T.: Blood picture of the experimental dengue infections in man and in mouse. Acta Scholae Medicinalis Universitatis in Kioto 30, 11—17 (1952).

HOTTA, S., YAMAMOTO, M., TOKUCHI, M., SAKAKIBARA, S.: Long persistence of anti-dengue antibodies in serum of native residents of Japanese Main Islands. Kobe J. med. Sci. 14, 149—153 (1968).

HOYLE, L.: The Influenza Viruses. (Virology Monographs, Vol. 4.) Wien-New York: Springer 1968.

IBRAHIM, A. N., HAMMON, W. McD.: Application of immunodiffusion methods to the antigenic analysis of dengue viruses. I. Precipitin-in-gel diffusion in two dimensions. J. Immunol. 100, 86—92 (1968a).

IBRAHIM, A. N., HAMMON, W. McD.: Application of immunodiffusion methods to the antigenic analysis of dengue viruses. II. Immunoelectrophoresis. J. Immunol. 100, 93—98 (1968b).

IBRAHIM, A. N., HAMMON, W. McD., POSTIC, B.: Cross plaque neutralization of two antigenically closely related dengue viruses (type 2 New Guinea C and TH-36). Proc. Soc. exp. Biol. (N.Y.) 128, 80—83 (1968c).

IGARASHI, A., MANTANI, M.: Rapid tritration of dengue virus type 4 infectivity by counting fluorescent foci. Biken J. 17, 87—93 (1974).

IGARASHI, A., STOLLAR, V.: Failure of defective interfering particles of Sindbis virus produced in BHK or chick cells to affect viral replication in A. albopictus cells J. Virol. 19, 398—408 (1976).

ISHII, N., YAJIMA, Y., MITOMA, Y.: Studies on dengue fever. III. Inoculation of dengue virus into the anterior chamber of the eye of rabbits. Nippon Igaku 3317, 156—158 (1943).

JOHNSON, K. M.: Further thoughts on arbovirus nomenclature. Amer. J. Epidem. 88, 305—306 (1968).

KATZ, L., PENMAN, J.: The solvent denaturation of double-stranded RNA from poliovirus infected HeLa cells. Biochem. biophys. Res. Commun. 23, 557—560 (1966).

KAWACHI, T.: Experiments on the inoculation of dengue virus into the anterior chamber of the eye of rabbits. Nippon Igaku 3343, 1340—1344 (1943).

KAWAMURA, R., FUKUSUMI, T., ITO, T., ITO, H., TAGAKI, S., OBATA, Y.: Cultivation of dengue virus, Rangoon type, in fertilized chick embryos. Nippon Igaku 3321, 335—342 (1943a).

KAWAMURA, R., FUKUSUMI, S., ITOH, T., ITOH, H., TAKAGI, S., OBATA, Y.: Kulturelle Ergebnisse im bebrüteten Hühnerei von Dengueerreger, Rangoon type. Kitasato Arch. exp. Med. 20, 1—26 (1943b).

KIMURA, R., HIGASHI, N., AKAZAWA, H.: Cultivation of dengue virus in fertilized chicken eggs. Nippon Igaku 3312, 2595—2599 (1942).

KIMURA, R., HIGASHI, N., AKAZAWA, H.: Über die Züchtung des Denguevirus auf der Chorioallantoismembran von Hühnereiern. Jap. J. med. Sci. 2, 241—246 (1944).

KIMURA, R., HOTTA, S.: On the inoculation of dengue virus into mice. Nippon Igaku **3379**, 629—633 (1944).

KOBAYASHI, E., TAKEDA, V., MORISHITA, K.: Inoculation of the etiologic agent of dengue into fertilized chicken eggs and brains of mice. Nippon Igaku **3319**, 241 to 244 (1943).

KOIZUMI, M., YAMAGUCHI, K., TONOMURA, K.: Dengue fever. Nisshin Igaku **6**, 955 to 1004 (1916).

KOKERNOT, R. H., SMITHBURN, K. C., WEINBREN, M. P.: Neutralizing antibodies to arthropod-borne viruses in human beings and animals in the Union of South Africa. J. Immunol. **77**, 313—323 (1956).

KONO, M.: Cultivation of dengue virus in fertilized chicken eggs. Gun-i-dan Zasshi (J. Milit. Surg. Japan) **358**, 259—272 (1942).

KOS, K. A., SHAPIRO, D., VAITUZIS, Z., RUSSELL, P. K.: Viral polypeptide composition of Japanese encephalitis virus-infected cell membranes. Arch. Virol. **47**, 217 to 224 (1975).

KUWAJIMA, Y., GOTO, J., HARA, T.: Experimental studies on dengue fever. I. Inoculation of the etiologic agent into the anterior chamber of the eye of rabbits. Nippon Igaku **3325**, 531—534 (1943).

LAM, K. S. K., MARSHALL, I. D.: Dual infections of *Aedes aegypti* with arboviruses. I. Arboviruses that have no apparent cytopathic effect in the mosquito. Amer. J. trop. Med. Hyg. **17**, 625—636 (1968).

LIEBHABER, H., GROSS, P. A.: The structural proteins of rubella virus. Virology **47**, 684—693 (1972).

LIKOSKY, W., CALISHER, C. H., MICHELSON, A. L., CORREA-CORONAS, R., HENDERSON, B. E., FELDMAN, R. A.: An epidemiologic study of dengue type 2 in Puerto Rico, 1969. Amer. J. Epidem. **97**, 264—275 (1973).

LUBINIECKI, A. S., TARR, G. C., HAMMON, W. McD.: Cloning of dengue virus type 2 by the direct fluorescent antibody techniques. Proc. Soc. exp. Biol. (N.Y.) **144**, 70—72 (1973).

LWOFF, A., TOURNIER, P.: The classification of viruses. Ann. Rev. Microbiol. **20**, 45—74 (1966).

MACKERRAS, I. M.: Transmission of dengue fever by *Aedes (Stegomyia) scutellaris* Walk. in New Guinea. Trans. roy. Soc. trop. Med. **40**, 295—312 (1946).

MAGUIRE, T., MILES, J. A. R.: The arbovirus carrier state in tissue cultures. Arch. ges. Virusforsch. **15**, 457—474 (1965).

MANOUSSAKIS, E.: Recherches étiologiques sur la dengue. Bull. Soc. Path. exot. **21**, 200—205 (1928).

MARCHETTE, N. J., HALSTEAD, S. B., FALKLER, W. A., JR., STENHOUSE, A., NASH, D.: Studies on the pathogenesis of dengue infection in monkeys. III. Sequential distribution of virus in primary and heterologous infections. J. infect. Dis. **128**, 23—30 (1973).

MATSUMURA, T., HOTTA, S. The characteristics of dengue virus hemagglutinin: An electron microscopic study. Virus **17**, 296—297 (1967).

MATSUMURA, T., HOTTA, S.: Electron microscopic observations on the purified dengue virus (type 1). Kobe J. med. Sci. **17**, 85—95 (1971).

MATSUMURA, T., SHIRAKI, K., HOTTA, S., SASHIKATA, T.: Release of arboviruses from cells cultivated with low ionic strength media. Proc. Soc. exp. Biol. (N.Y.) **141**, 599—605 (1972b).

MATSUMURA, T., STOLLAR, V., SCHLESINGER, R. W.: Studies on the nature of dengue viruses. V. Structure and development of dengue virus in Vero cells. Virology **46**, 344—355 (1971).

MATSUMURA, T., STOLLAR, V., SCHLESINGER, R. W.: Effects of ionic strength on the release of dengue virus from Vero cells. J. gen. Virol. **17**, 343—347 (1972a).

MATSUMURA, T., TAKEHARA, M., HOTTA, S.: Some fundamental characteristics of dengue and yellow fever viruses; inhomogeneity and characterization of partially purified viral particles. Kobe J. med. Sci. **13**, 273—293 (1967).

MATTINGLY, P. F.: Symposium on the evolution of arbovirus diseases. II. Ecological aspects of the evolution of mosquito-borne virus diseases. Trans. roy. Soc. trop. Med. Hyg. 54, 97—112 (1960).

McCLOUD, T. G., CARDIFF, R. D., BRANDT, W. E., CHIEWSILP, D., RUSSELL, P. K.: Separation of dengue strains on the basis of a nonstructural antigen. Amer. J. trop. Med. Hyg. 20, 964—968 (1971).

McCoy, O. R.: Dengue, Part I. Epidemiologic considerations. Chapter IV in "Preventive Medicine in World War II, Vol. VII, Communicable Diseases" (COATES, HOFF, eds.), pp. 29—40. Washington, D.C.: Office of the Surgeon General, Department of the Army 1964.

McLEAN, D. M., CLARKE, A. M., COLEMAN, J. C., MONTALBETTI, C. A., SKIDMORE, A. G., WALTERS, T. E., WISE, R.: Vector capability of Aedes aegypti mosquitoes for California encephalitis and dengue viruses at various temperatures. Canad. J. Microbiol. 20, 255—262 (1974).

MEIKLEJOHN, G., ENGLAND, B., LENNETTE, E. H.: Propagation of dengue virus strains in unweaned mice. Amer. J. trop. Med. Hyg. 1, 51—58 (1952a).

MEIKLEJOHN, G., ENGLAND, B., LENNETTE, E. H.: Adaptation of dengue virus to the hamster. Amer. J. trop. Med. Hyg. 1, 59—65 (1952b).

MELNICK, J. L.: Classification and nomenclature of viruses, 1973. Progr. med. Virol. 16, 337—342 (1973).

METTLER, N. E., PETRELLI, R. L., CASALS, J.: Absence of antigenic cross-reactions between rubella virus and arboviruses. Virology 36, 503—504 (1968).

MILES, J. A. R., AUSTIN, F. J.: The formation of plaques in tissue culture by arboviruses. Aust. J. exp. Biol. med. Sci. 41, 199—204 (1963).

MILLER, H. K., SCHLESINGER, R. W.: Differentiation and purification of influenza viruses by adsorption and aluminum phosphate. J. Immunol. 75, 155—160 (1955).

MISAO, T., KANEHISA, T., YAMADA, H., ETO, H., HARADA, Y.: Studies on dengue fever. X. Inoculation of dengue virus into monkeys (clinical aspects). Rinsho & Kenkyu (Clinic & Research) 23, 401—405 (1946a).

MISAO, T., KANEHISA, T., YAMADA, H., ETO, H., HARADA, Y., SAKANE, H., SHIRAISHI, T.: Studies on dengue fever. XI. Inoculation of dengue virus into monkeys (Pathological aspects). Rinsho & Kenkyu (Clinic & Research) 23, 527—533 (1946b).

MISAO, T., YAMAOKA, K., YAMADA, Y., MITSUNO, T., KOIWAI, R., ICHINOSE, J., IWAKURA, G., KUSHIMOTO, G.: Cultivation of dengue virus in fertilized chicken eggs. Nippon Igaku 3321, 343—344 (1943).

MORALES, A., GROOT, H., RUSSELL, P. K., McCOWN, J. M.: Recovery of dengue-2 virus from Aedes aegypti in Columbia. Amer. J. trop. Med. Hyg. 22, 785—787 (1973).

MOREAU, J. P., ROSEN, L., SAUGRAIN, J., LAGRAULET, J.: An epidemic of dengue on Tahiti associated with hemorrhagic manifestations. Amer. J. trop. Med. Hyg. 22, 237—241 (1973).

MURPHY, F. A., HARRISON, A. K., WHITFIELD, S. G., Bunyaviridae: Morphologic and morphogenetic similarities of Bunyamwera supergroup viruses and several other arthropod-borne viruses. Intervirology 1, 297—316 (1973)

MYERS, R. M., CAREY, D. E., REUBEN, R., JESUDASS, E., RANITZ, C. D. S., JADHAV, M.: The 1964 epidemic of dengue-like fever in South India: Isolation of chikungunya virus from human sera and from mosquitoes. Indian J. med. Res. 53, 1—8 (1965).

NAKAGAWA, Y.: Purification of dengue virus. Virus 3, 6—11 (1953).

NAKAGAWA, Y., SHINGU, M.: Purification of dengue virus: Morphological observations of purified dengue virus by electron microscopy. Virus 7, 190—198 (1957).

NAKAGAWA, Y., SHINGU, M.: Inoculation of dengue virus in one-day-old hen's egg. Virus 8, 118—120 (1958).

NAKAGAWA, Y., SHINGU, M.: Studies on hemagglutination with dengue virus. I. Conditions and properties of hemagglutination. Kurume med. J. 2, 157—165 (1955).

NAKAMURA, M.: Infectious ribonucleic acid derived from mouse brains infected with two kinds of arbovirus group B. Nature (Lond.) 191, 624 (1961).

NATHANSON, N., DAVIS, M., THIND. I. S., PRICE, W. H.: Histological studies of the monkey neurovirulence of group B arboviruses. II. Selection of indicator centers. Amer. J. Epidem. **84**, 524—540 (1966).

NATHANSON, N., GITTELSOHN, A. M., THIND, I. S., PRICE, W. H.: Histological studies of the monkey neurovirulence of group B arboviruses. III. Relative virulence of selected viruses. Amer. J. Epidem. **83**, 503—517 (1967).

NATHANSON, N., GOLDBLATT, D., THIND, I. S., DAVIS, M., PRICE. W. H.: Histological studies of the monkey neurovirulence of group B arboviruses. I. A semiquantitative grading scale. Amer. J. Epidem. **82**, 359—381 (1965).

NEFF, J. M., MORRIS, L., GONZALES-ALCOVER, R., COLEMAN, P. H., LYSS, S. B., NEGRON, H.: Dengue fever in a Puerto Rican community. Amer. J. Epidem. **86**, 162—184 (1967).

NIMMANNITYA, S., HALSTEAD, S. B., COHEN, S. N., MARGIOTTA, M. R.: Dengue and chikungunya virus infection in man in Thailand, 1962—1964. I. Observations on hospitalized patients with hemorrhagic fever. Amer. J. trop. Med. Hyg. **18**, 954—971 (1969).

NISALAK, A., HALSTEAD, S. B., SINGHARAT, P., UDOMSAKDI, S., NYE, S. W., VINIJCHAIKUL, K.: Observations related to pathogenesis of dengue hemorrhagic fever. III. Virologic studies of fatal disease. Yale J. Biol. Med. **42**, 293—310 (1970).

OGATA, N., HASHIMOTO, H.: *In vitro* survival time and preservation of dengue virus. Nippon Igaku **3379**, 639—641 (1944a).

OGATA, N., HASHIMOTO, H.: Animal inoculation of dengue virus and inapparent infection thereof. Nippon Igaku **3379**, 641—644 (1944b).

OGATA, N., YOSHII, M.: Isolation, preservation and characterization of dengue virus. Nippon Igaku **3338**, 1124—1128 (1943).

OHTAKA, Y., SPIEGELMAN, S.: Translational control of protein synthesis in a cell-free system directed by polycistronic viral RNA. Science **142**, 493—497 (1963).

OHYAMA, A., IGARASHI, A., MANTANI, M., NAITO, T., TUCHINDA, P., FUKAI, K.: Morphological studies on dengue virus infected cells. Virus **17**, 316—317 (1967).

OSGOOD, D.: Remarks on the dengue. Boston med. surg. J. **1**, 561—563 (1828).

OTAWARA, T., ROKUTANDA, T., TAKAYAMA, Y., KUSUDA, K., ITSUNO, T., OGURI, K., KANEMITSU, M., ITO, K., KOTAKE, K.: Studies on dengue fever. I. Inoculation of dengue virus into monkeys. Nippon Igaku **3326**, 575—578 (1943).

OZAWA, Y.: Studies on dengue fever virus by electron microscopy. Yokohama med. Bull. **5**, 72—75 (1954).

PAUL, J. R., MELNICK, J. L., SABIN, A. B.: Experimental attempts to transmit phlebotomus (sandfly, pappataci) and dengue fevers to chimpanzees. Proc. Soc. exp. Biol. (N.Y.) **68**, 193—198 (1948).

PAUL, S. D.: Comparative susceptibility of primary cultures from renal epithelial cells of *Macaca radiata* and BS-C-1 cell line for the isolation of dengue viruses. Indian J. med. Res. **56**, 142—149 (1968).

PAUL, S. D., BANERJEE, K.: Adaptation of freshly isolated strains of dengue virus to tissue culture. Indian J. med. Res. **53**, 405—409 (1965).

PAUL, S. D., SINGH, K. R. P.: Comparative sensitivity of mosquito cell lines, Vero cell lines, and infant mice to infection with arboviruses. Curr. Sci. **38**, 241—242 (1969).

PAUL, S. D., SINGH, K. R. P., BHAT, U. K. M.: A study of the cytopathic effect of arboviruses on cultures from *Aedes albopictus* cell line. Indian J. med. Res. **57**, 339 to 348 (1969).

PAVLATOS, M., SMITH, C. E. G.: Antibodies to arthropod-borne viruses in Greece. Trans. roy. Soc. trop. Med. Hyg. **58**, 422—424 (1964).

PELEG, J.: Attenuation of Semliki Forest (SF) virus in continuously cultured *Aedes aegypti* mosquito cells (Peleg) as a step in production of vaccines. Curr. Top. Microbiol. Immunol. **55**, 155—164 (1971).

PELEG, J., STOLLAR, V.: Homologous interference in *Aedes aegypti* cell cultures infected with Sindbis virus. Arch. ges. Virusforsch. **45**, 309—318 (1974).

PFEFFERKORN, E.: Arboviruses and vesicular stomatitis virus. In: Molecular Basis of Virology, ACS Monograph (FRAENKEL-CONRAT, H., ed.), pp. 332—350. New York: Reinhold Book Corp. 1968.

PFEFFERKORN, E. R., SHAPIRO, D.: Reproduction of Togaviruses. In: Comprehensive Virology (FRAENKEL-CONRAT, H., WAGNER, R. R., eds.), Vol. 2, pp. 171—230. New York-London: Plenum Press 1974.

POND, W. L., EHRENKRANZ, N. J., DANAUSKAS, J. X., CARTER, M. J.: Heterotypic serological responses after yellow fever vaccination; detection of persons with past St. Louis encephalitis or dengue. J. Immunol. 98, 673—682 (1967).

POND, W. L., EHRENKRANZ, N. J., DANAUSKAS, J. X., DAVIES, J. E.: Arboviruses and human disease in South Florida. Amer. J. trop. Med. Hyg. 15, 205—210 (1966).

PORTERFIELD, J. S.: Use of goose cells in haemagglutination tests with arthropod-borne viruses. Nature (Lond.) 180, 1201—1202 (1957).

PORTERFIELD, J. S., CASALS, J., CHUMAKOV, M. P., GAIDAMOVICH, S. Y., HANNOUN, C., HOLMES, I. H., HORZINEK, M. C., MUSSGAY, M., RUSSELL, P. K.: Bunyaviruses and Bunyaviridae. Intervirology 2, 270—272 (1974).

PRICE, W. H., CASALS, J., O'LEARY, W.: Studies on the sequential immunization against group B arboviruses in squirrel monkeys, cynomolgus monkeys and chimpanzees. Amer. J. trop. Med. Hyg. 23, 118 (1974).

PRICE, W. H., CASALS, J., THIND, I., O'LEARY, W.: Sequential immunization procedures using living attenuated 17 D yellow fever virus, living attenuated Langat E5 virus, and living attenuated dengue 2 virus (New Guinea C Isolate). Amer. J. trop. Med. Hyg. 22, 509—523 (1973 a).

PRICE, W. H., THIND, I. S.: The mechanism of cross-protection afforded by dengue virus against West Nile virus in hamsters. J. Hyg. (Lond.) 70, 611—617 (1972).

PRICE, W. H., THIND, I. S., O'LEARY, W.: The attenuation of the 26th mouse brain passage of New Guinea C strain of dengue 2 virus for use in the sequential immunization procedure against group B arboviruses. Amer. J. trop. Med. Hyg. 22, 92—99 (1973 b).

QURESHI, A. A., TRENT, D. W.: Group B arbovirus structural and nonstructural antigens. II. Purification of Saint Louis encephalitis virus intracellular antigens. Infect. & Immun. 8, 985—992 (1973).

QURESHI, A. A., TRENT, D. W.: Group B arbovirus structural and nonstructural antigens. III. Serological specificity of solubilized intracellular viral proteins. Infect. & Immun. 8, 993—999 (1973).

REAGAN, R. L., BRUECKNER, A. L.: Studies of dengue fever virus by electron microscopy. J. Bact. 64, 233—235 (1952 a).

REAGAN, R. L., BRUECKNER, A. L.: Studies of dengue fever virus in the cave bat (Myotus lucifugus). J. infect. Dis. 91, 145—146 (1952 b).

REED, L. J., MUENCH, H.: A simple method of estimating fifty percent endpoints. Amer. J. Hyg. 27, 493—497 (1938).

REUL, R., ERRAERTS, W.: Une épidémie de "dengue-like fever" dans la province de l'équateur au Congo Belge. Ann. Soc. belge Méd. trop. 29, 151—175 (1949).

ROSATO, R. R., DALRYMPLE, J. M., BRANDT, W. E., CARDIFF, R. D., RUSSELL, P. K.: Biophysical separation of major arbovirus subgroups. Acta virol. 18, 25—30 (1974).

ROSEN, L.: Experimental infection of new world monkeys with dengue and yellow fever viruses. Amer. J. trop. Med. Hyg. 7, 406—410 (1958).

ROSEN, L.: A recent outbreak of dengue in French Polynesia. Jap. J. med. Sci. Biol. 20 (Suppl.), 67—69 (1967).

ROSEN, L., GUBLER, D.: The use of mosquitoes to detect and propagate dengue viruses. Amer. J. trop. Med. Hyg. 23, 1153—1160 (1974).

ROSEN, L., ROZEBOOM, L. E., SWEET, B. H., SABIN, A. B.: The transmission of dengue by Aedes polynesiensis Marks. Amer. J. trop. Med. Hyg. 3, 878—882 (1954).

RUDNICK, A.: Studies of the ecology of dengue in Malaysia. Bull. Wld Hlth Org. 35, 78—79 (1966). Also: J. med. Entomol. 2, 203—208 (1965).

RUDNICK, A., CHAN, Y. C.: Dengue type 2 virus in naturally infected Aedes albopictus mosquitoes in Singapore. Science 149, 638—639 (1965).

RUSSELL, P. K.: Pathogenesis of the dengue shock syndrome: evidence for an immuno-logic mechanism. In: Immunopathology, 6th Int. Symposium (MIESCHER, P. A., ed.), pp. 426—435. Basel-Stuttgart: Schwabe and Co. 1970.

RUSSELL, P. K.: Immunopathologic mechanisms in the dengue shock syndrome. In: Progress in Immunology (AMOS, B., ed.), pp. 831—838. New York: Academic Press 1971.

RUSSELL, P. K., BELLANTI, J. A., BUESCHER, E. L., McCOWN, J. M.: Challenge virus resistance and interferon produced in BS-C-1 cells by dengue virus. Proc. Soc. exp. Biol. (N.Y.) 122, 557—561 (1966a).

RUSSELL, P. K., BUESCHER, E. L., McCOWN, J. M., ORDONEZ, J.: Recovery of dengue viruses from patients during epidemics in Puerto Rico and East Pakistan. Amer. J. trop. Med. Hyg. 15, 573—579 (1966b).

RUSSELL, P. K., BRANDT, W. E.: Immunopathologic processes and viral antigens associated with sequential dengue virus infection. In: Perspectives in Virology, Vol. VIII, pp. 263—277. New York-London: Academic Press 1973.

RUSSELL, P. K., CHIEWSILP, D., BRANDT, W. E.: Immunoprecipitation analysis of soluble complement-fixing antigens of dengue viruses. J. Immunol. 105, 838—845 (1970).

RUSSELL, P. K., CHUMDERMPADETSUK, S., PIYARATN, P.: A fatal case of dengue hemorrhagic fever in an American child. Pediatrics 40, 804—807 (1967).

RUSSELL, P. K., GOULD, D. J., YUILL, T. M., NISALAK, A., WINTER, P. E.: Recovery of dengue-4 viruses from mosquito vectors and patients during an epidemic of dengue hemorrhagic fever. Amer. J. trop. Med. Hyg. 18, 580—583 (1969).

RUSSELL, P. K., INTAVIVAT, A., KANCHANAPILANT, S.: Anti-dengue immunoglobulins and serum β_1 c/a globulin levels in dengue shock syndrome. J. Immunol. 102, 412 to 420 (1969).

RUSSELL, P. K., McCOWN, J. M.: Comparison of dengue-2 and dengue-3 virus strains by neutralization tests and identification of a subtype of dengue-3. Amer. J. trop. Med. Hyg. 21, 97—99 (1972).

RUSSELL, P. K., NISALAK, A.: Dengue virus identification by the plaque reduction neutralization test. J. Immunol. 99, 291—296 (1967).

RUSSELL, P. K., NISALAK, A., SUKHAVACHANA, P., VIVONA, S.: A plaque reduction test for dengue virus neutralizing antibodies. J. Immunol. 99, 285—290 (1967).

RUSSELL, P. K., QUY, D. V., NISALAK, A., SIMASTHIEN, P., YUILL, T. M., GOULD, D. J.: Mosquito vectors of dengue viruses in South Vietnam. Amer. J. trop. Med. Hyg. 18, 455—459 (1969b).

RUSSELL, P. K., YUILL, T. M., NISALAK, A., UDOMSAKDI, S., GOULD, D. J., WINTER, P. E.: An insular outbreak of dengue hemorrhagic fever. II. Virologic and serologic studies. Amer. J. trop. Med. Hyg. 17, 600—608 (1968).

SABIN, A. B.: Dengue. In: Viral and Rickettsial Infections of Man (RIVERS, T. M., ed.), pp. 445—453. Philadelphia: Lippincott 1948a.

SABIN, A. B.: Dengue. In: Diagnostic Procedures for Virus and Rickettsial Diseases, 1st ed., pp. 289—293. Amer. publ. Hlth Assn. 1948b.

SABIN, A. B.: Recent advances in phlebotomus and dengue fevers. Proc. 4th Int. Congr. trop. Med. & Malaria, Washington, D.C., May 10—18, 1948, pp. 520—525 (1948c).

SABIN, A. B.: The dengue group of viruses and its family relationships. Bact. Rev. 14, 225—232 (1950).

SABIN, A. B.: Research on dengue during World War II. Amer. J. trop. Med. Hyg. 1, 30—50 (1952a).

SABIN, A. B.: Genetic, hormonal and age factors in natural resistance to certain viruses. Ann. N.Y. Acad. Sci. 54, 936—944 (1952b).

SABIN, A. B.: Nature of inherited resistance to viruses affecting the nervous system. Proc. nat. Acad. Sci. (Wash.) 38, 540—546 (1952c).

SABIN, A. B.: Dengue. In: Viral and Rickettsial Infections of Man, 2nd ed. (RIVERS, T. M., ed.), pp. 556—568. Philadelphia: Lippincott 1952d.

SABIN, A. B.: Genetic factors affecting susceptibility and resistance to virus disease of the nervous system. Proc. Assn. for Research in Nervous and Mental Disease, Vol. XXXIII, pp. 57—66 (1954).

SABIN, A. B.: Recent advances in our knowledge of dengue and sandfly fever. Amer. J. trop. Med. Hyg. 4, 198—207 (1955).

SABIN, A. B.: Dengue. In: Viral and Rickettsial Infections of Man (RIVERS, T. M., HORSFALL, F. L., JR., eds.), pp. 361—373. Philadelphia: Lippincott 1959.

SABIN, A. B., SCHLESINGER, R. W.: Production of immunity to dengue with virus modified by propagation in mice. Science 101, 640—642 (1945).

SABIN, A. B., THEILER, M.: Interference between the viruses of dengue and yellow fever. Cited from SABIN, A. B. (1948a) (1944).

SABIN, A. B., YOUNG, I.: A complement fixation test for dengue. Proc. Soc. exp. Biol. (N.Y.) 69, 478—480 (1949).

SALK, J. E.: A simplified procedure for titrating hemagglutinating capacity of influenza-virus and the corresponding antibody. J. Immunol. 49, 87—98 (1944).

SARTORELLI, A. C., FISCHER, D. S., DOWNS, W. G.: Use of sarcoma 180/TG to prepare hyperimmune ascitic fluid in the mouse. J. Immunol. 96, 676 (1965).

SCHERER, W. F.: The complexity of arbovirus nomenclature; a proposal to simplify it. Amer. J. Epidem. 88, 145—146 (1968).

SCHERER, W. F., BREAKENRIDGE, F. A., DICKERMAN, R. W.: Cross-protection studies and search for subclinical disease in New World monkeys infected sequentially with different immunologic types of dengue virus. Amer. J. Epidem. 95, 67—79 (1972).

SCHLESINGER, M. J., SCHLESINGER, S., BURGE, B. W.: Identification of a second glyco-protein in Sindbis virus. Virology 47, 539—541 (1972).

SCHLESINGER, R. W.: Propagation in chick embryos of the Hawaiian strain of dengue virus. I. Sustained serial passage in eggs after one hundred and one intracerebral passages in mice. Amer. J. Hyg. 51, 248—254 (1950).

SCHLESINGER, R. W.: Propagation in chick embryos of dengue virus, Hawaiian strain. II. Findings in infected eggs. Proc. Soc. exp. Biol. (N.Y.) 76, 817—823 (1951).

SCHLESINGER, R. W.: Dengue. In: A Textbook of Medicine, 10th ed. (CECIL, R. L., LOEB, R. F., eds.), pp. 14—16. Philadelphia: W. B. Saunders Co. 1958.

SCHLESINGER, R. W.: New opportunities in biological research offered by arthropod cell cultures. I. Some speculations on the possible role of arthropods in the evolution of arboviruses. In: Curr. Top. Microbiol. Immunol. 55, pp. 241—245. Berlin-Heidelberg-New York: Springer 1971.

SCHLESINGER, R. W.: Sindbis virus replication in vertebrate and mosquito cells: An interpretation. Medical Biology 53, 295—301 (1975).

SCHLESINGER, R. W., FRANKEL, J. W.: Adaptation of the "New Guinea B" strain of dengue virus to suckling and to adult Swiss mice: A study in viral variation. Amer. J. trop. Med. Hyg. 1, 66—77 (1952a).

SCHLESINGER, R. W., FRANKEL, J. W.: Interference as a factor in the adaptation to mice of a strain of dengue virus. Bact. Proc., p. 85 (1952b).

SCHLESINGER, R. W., GORDON, I., FRANKEL, J. W., WINTER, J. W., PATTERSON, P. R., DORRANCE, W. R.: Clinical and serologic response of man to immunization with attenuated dengue and yellow fever viruses. J. Immunol. 77, 352—364 (1956).

SCHLESINGER, S., SCHLESINGER, M. J.: Formation of Sindbis virus proteins: Identifica-tion of a precursor for one of the envelope proteins. J. Virol. 10, 925—932 (1972).

SCHULZE, I. T.: Experimental studies on dengue virus. Ph.D. Thesis, St. Louis University, 1962.

SCHULZE, I. T.: Reversible inhibition of type 2 dengue virus by agar polysaccharide. Virology 22, 79—90 (1964).

SCHULZE, I. T.: Structure of the influenza virion. Advanc. Virus Res. 18, 1—55 (1973).

SCHULZE, I. T., SCHLESINGER, R. W.: Plaque assay of dengue and other group B arthropod-borne viruses under methyl cellulose overlay media. Virology 19, 40—48 (1963a).

SCHULZE, I. T., SCHLESINGER. R. W.: Inhibition of infectious and hemagglutinating properties of type 2 dengue virus by aqueous agar extracts. Virology **19**. 49—57 (1963b).

SCOTT, R. M., McCOWN, J. M., RUSSELL, P. K.: Human immunoglobulins specificity after group B arbovirus infections. Infect. & Immun. **6**, 277—281 (1972).

SCOTT, R. M., RUSSELL, P. K.: Complement fixation blocking activity of anti-dengue IgM antibody. J. Immunol. **109**, 875—877 (1972).

SHAPIRO, D., BRANDT, W. E., CARDIFF, R. D., RUSSELL, P. K.: The proteins of Japanese encephalitis virus. Virology **44**, 108—124 (1971).

SHAPIRO, D., BRANDT, W. E., RUSSELL. P. K.: Change involving a viral membrane glycoprotein during morphogenesis of group B arboviruses. Virology **50**, 906—911 (1972b).

SHAPIRO, D., KOS, K., BRANDT, W. E., RUSSELL, P. K.: Membrane-bound proteins of Japanese encephalitis virus-infected chick embryo cells. Virology **48**, 360—372 (1972c).

SHAPIRO, D., KOS, K., RUSSELL, P. K.: Japanese encephalitis virus glycoproteins. Virology **56**, 88—94 (1973a).

SHAPIRO, D., KOS, K., RUSSELL, P. K.: Protein synthesis in Japanese encephalitis virus-infected cells. Virology **56**, 95—109 (1973b).

SHAPIRO, D., TRENT, D., BRANDT, W. E., RUSSELL, P. K.: Comparison of the virion polypeptides of group B arboviruses. Infect. & Immun. **6**, 206—209 (1972d).

SHENK, T. E., KOSHELNYK, K. A., STOLLAR, V.: Temperature-sensitive virus from *Aedes albopictus* cells chronically infected with Sindbis virus. J. Virol. **13**, 439—447 (1974).

SHIMAZU, Y., AOKI, H., HOTTA, S.: Research on dengue in tissue culture. II. Further observations on virus-tissue culture affinity. Kobe J. med. Sci. **12**, 189—198 (1966).

SHINGU. M.: Studies on hemagglutination by dengue virus. I. The conditions and specific properties of hemagglutination reaction. Virus **5**, 230—241 (1955).

SHINGU, M.: Studies on hemagglutination by dengue virus. II. The properties of hemagglutination and the role of calcium chloride in the hemagglutination. Virus **6**, 442—453 (1956).

SHORTT, H. E., RAO, R. S., SWAMINATH, C. S.: Cultivation of the viruses of sandfly fever on the chorio-allantoic membrane of the chick embryo. Indian J. med. Res. **23**, 865—870 (1936).

SIGEL, M. M., BEASLEY, A. R.: Studies on dengue fever. Tex. Rep. Biol. Med. **17**, 618—623 (1959).

SILER, J. F., HALL, M. W., HITCHENS, A. P.: Dengue: Its history, epidemiology, mechanism of transmission, etiology, clinical manifestations, immunity and prevention. Philipp. J. Sci. **29**, 1—304 (1926).

SIMMONS, D. T., STRAUSS, J. H.: Replication of Sindbis virus. I. Relative size and genetic content of 26S and 49S RNA. J. molec. Biol. **71**, 599—613 (1972).

SIMMONS, J. S., ST. JOHN, J. H., REYNOLDS, F. H. K.: Experimental studies of dengue. Philipp. J. Sci. **44**, 1—247 (1931).

SINARACHATANANT, P., OLSON, L. C.: Replication of dengue virus type 2 in *Aedes albopictus* cell culture. J. Virol. **12**, 275—283 (1973).

SINGH, K. R. P.: Cell cultures derived from larvae of *Aedes albopictus* (Skuse) and *Aedes aegypti* (L.). Curr. Sci. **36**, 506—508 (1967).

SINGH, K. R. P.: Growth of arboviruses in *Aedes albopictus* and *A. aegypti* cell lines. Curr. Top. Microbiol. Immunol. **55**, 127—133 (1971).

SINGH, K. R. P., PAUL, S. D.: Multiplication of arboviruses in cell lines from *Aedes albopictus* and *Aedes aegypti*. Curr. Sci. **37**, 65—67 (1968).

SINGH, K. R. P., PAUL, S. D.: Isolation of dengue viruses in *Aedes albopictus* cell cultures. Bull. Wld Hlth Org. **40**, 982—983 (1969).

SMITH, C. E. G.: Isolation of three strains of type 1 dengue virus from a local outbreak of the disease in Malaya. J. Hyg. (Lond.) **54**, 569—580 (1956).

SMITH, C. E. G., WESTGARTH, D. R.: The use of survival time in the analysis of neutralization tests for serum antibody surveys. J. Hyg. (Lond.) **55**, 224—238 (1957).

SMITH, T. J., BRANDT, W. E., SWANSON, J. L., McCOWN, J. M., BUESCHER, E. L.: Physical and biological properties of dengue-2 virus and associated antigens. J. Virol. **5**, 524—532 (1970).

SMITH, T. J., WINTER, P. E., NISALAK, A., UDOMSAKDI, S.: Dengue control on an Island in the Gulf of Thailand. II. Virological studies. Amer. J. trop. Med. Hyg. **20**, 715—719 (1971).

SMITHBURN, K. C.: Antigenic relationships among certain arthropod-borne viruses as revealed by neutralization tests. J. Immunol. **72**, 376—388 (1954).

SPENCE, L., JONKERS, A. H., CASALS, J.: Dengue type 3 virus isolated from an Antiguan patient during the 1963—64 Caribbean epidemic. Amer. J. trop. Med. Hyg. **18**, 584—587 (1969).

SRIURAIRATNA, S., BHAMARAPRATI, N., PHALAVADHTANA, O.: Dengue virus infection of mice: morphology and morphogenesis of dengue type-2 virus in suckling mouse neurones. Infect. & Immun. **8**, 1017—1028 (1973).

STEVENS, T. M.: Arbovirus replication in mosquito cell lines (Singh) grown in monolayer or suspension culture. Proc. Soc. exp. Biol. (N.Y.) **134**, 356—361 (1970).

STEVENS, T. M., SCHLESINGER, R. W.: Characterization of dengue virus. Fed. Proc. **22**, 674 (1963) (Abstract).

STEVENS, T. M., SCHLESINGER, R. W.: Studies on the nature of dengue viruses. I. Correlation of particle density, infectivity, and RNA content of type 2 virus. Virology **27**, 103—112 (1965).

STEVENS, T. M., SCHLESINGER, R. W., SCHULZE, I. T.: Concurrent increase of plaque-forming and hemagglutinating activities during growth of dengue virus in KB cells. Bact. Proc., p. 132 (1962) (Abstract).

STEWART, F. H.: Dengue: Analysis of the clinical syndrome at a South Pacific advance base. U.S. Naval med. Bull. **42**, 1233—1240 (1944).

STIM, T. B.: Arbovirus plaquing in two simian kidney cell lines. J. gen. Virol. **5**, 329 to 338 (1969).

STIM, T. B.: Dengue virus plaque development in Simian cell systems. I. Factors influencing virus adsorption and variables in the agar overlay medium. Appl. Microbiol. **19**, 751—756 (1970a).

STIM, T. B.: Dengue virus plaque development in Simian cell systems. II. Agar variables in effect of chemical additives. Appl. Microbiol. **19**, 757—762 (1970b).

STIM, T. B., HENDERSON, J. R.: Further studies on multiplication of dengue viruses in various host systems. Proc. Soc. exp. Biol. (N.Y.) **122**, 1004 (1966).

STOHLMAN, S. A., WISSEMAN, C. L., JR., EYLAR, O. R., SILVERMAN, D. J.: Dengue virus-induced modifications of host cell membranes. J. Virol. **16**, 1017—1026 (1975).

STOLLAR, B. D., STOLLAR, V.: Immunofluorescent demonstration of double-stranded RNA in the cytoplasm of Sindbis virus-infected cells. Virology **42**, 276—280 (1970b).

STOLLAR, V.: Studies on the nature of dengue viruses. IV. The structural proteins of type 2 dengue virus. Virology **39**, 426—438 (1969).

STOLLAR, V.: Immune lysis of Sindbis virus. Virology **66**, 620—624 (1975).

STOLLAR, V., PELEG, J., SHENK, T. E.: Temperature sensitivity of a Sindbis virus mutant isolated from persistently infected *Aedes aegypti* cell culture. Intervirology **2**, 337—344 (1974).

STOLLAR, V., SCHLESINGER, R. W., STEVENS, T. M.: Studies on the nature of dengue viruses. III. RNA synthesis in cells infected with type 2 dengue virus. Virology **33**, 650—658 (1967).

STOLLAR, V., SHENK, T. E.: Homologous viral interference in *Aedes albopictus* cultures chronically infected with Sindbis virus. J. Virol. **11**, 592—595 (1973).

STOLLAR, V., STEVENS, T. M., SCHLESINGER, R. W.: Studies on the nature of dengue viruses. II. Characterization of viral RNA and effects of inhibitors of RNA synthesis. Virology **30**, 303—312 (1966).

STOLLAR, V., STOLLAR, B. D.: Immunochemical measurement of double-stranded RNA of uninfected and arbovirus-infected mammalian cells. Proc. nat. Acad. Sci. (Wash.) **65**, 993—1000 (1970a).

STOLLAR, V., STOLLAR, B. D., KOO, R., HARRAP, K. A., SCHLESINGER, R. W.: Sialic acid contents of Sindbis virus from vertebrate and mosquito cells: Equivalence of biological and immunological viral properties. Virology **69**, 104—115 (1976).

STRAUSS, T. H., BURGE, B. W., DARNELL, J. E.: Sindbis virus infection of chick and hamster cells: Synthesis of virus specific proteins. Virology **37**, 367—376 (1969).

STRAUSS, T. H., BURGE, B. W., DARNELL, J. E.: Carbohydrate content of the membrane protein of Sindbis virus. J. molec. Biol. **47**, 437—448 (1970).

STRAUSS, T. H., BURGE, B. W., PFEFFERKORN, E. R., DARNELL, J. E.: Identification of the membrane protein and "core" protein of Sindbis virus. Proc. nat. Acad. Sci. (Wash.) **599**, 533—537 (1968).

STRODE, G. K., BUGHER, J. C., KERR, J. A., SMITH, H. H'., SMITHBURN, K. C., TAYLOR, R. M., THEILER, M., WARREN, A. J., WHITMAN, L. (eds.). In: Yellow Fever. New York: McGraw-Hill 1951.

SUITOR, E. C., JR., PAUL, F. L.: Syncytia formation of mosquito cell cultures mediated by type 2 dengue virus. Virology **38**, 482—483 (1969).

SUKHAVACHANA, P., NISALAK, A., HALSTEAD, S. B.: Tissue culture techniques for the study of dengue viruses. Bull. Wld Hlth Org. **35**, 65 (1966).

SUMMERS, D. F., MAIZEL, J. V., JR., DARNELL, J. E., JR.: Evidence for virus-specific noncapsid proteins in poliovirus-infected HeLa cells. Proc. nat. Acad. Sci. (Wash.) **54**, 505—513 (1965).

SUNG, J. S., DIWAN, A. R., FALKLER, W. A., JR., YANG, H. Y., HALSTEAD, S. B.: Dengue carrier culture and antigen production in human lymphoblastoid lines. Intervirology **5**, 137—149 (1975).

SWEET, B. H., HATGI, J., POLISE, F.: Experimental infection of African green monkeys with unadapted type 1 dengue virus by the incutaneous and oral routes. Bact. Proc. p. 160 (1969).

SWEET, B. H., SABIN, A. B.: Properties and antigenic relationships of hemagglutinins associated with the dengue viruses. J. Immunol. **73**, 363—373 (1954a).

SWEET, B. H., UTHANK, H. D.: A comparative study of viral susceptibility of monolayers and suspended mosquito cell lines. Curr. Top. Microbiol. Immunol. **55**, 150—154 (1971).

TAKEHARA, M., HOTTA, S.: Effect of enzymes on partially purified Japanese B encephalitis and related arboviruses. Science **134**, 1878—1880 (1961).

TANIGUCHI, T.: Etiology and immunity of dengue fever: Studies on animal inoculation and cultivation. Report, Japanese Army Medical School, Part II, No. 632, pp. 1—49 (1943).

TANIGUCHI, T., FUJINO, T., INOKI, S., OKUNO, Y.: Studies on the experimental inoculation of dengue fever. Med. J. Osaka Univ. **2**, 1—36 (1951).

TARR, G. C., HAMMON, W. McD.: Cross-protection between group B arboviruses: Resistance in mice to Japanese B encephalitis and St. Louis encephalitis viruses induced by dengue virus immunization. Infect. & Immun. **9**, 909—915 (1974).

TARR, G. C., LUBINIECKI, A. S.: Chemically induced temperature-sensitive mutants of dengue virus type 2: Comparison of temperature sensitivity *in vitro* with infectivity in suckling mice, hamsters, and rhesus monkeys. Infect. & Immun. **13**, 688—695 (1976).

TAURASO, N. M., SHELOKOV, A.: Arboviruses: A problem in classification. Arch. ges. Virusforsch. **22**, 273—279 (1967).

TAYLOR, R. M. (ed.): Arthropod-borne viruses. Report of a study group, Wld Hlth Org. techn. Rep. Ser. **219**, 1—68 (1961).

THEILER, M.: Action of sodium desoxycholate on arthropod-borne viruses. Proc. Soc. exp. Biol. (N.Y.) **96**, 380—382 (1957).

THEILER, M., ANDERSON, C. R.: The relative resistance of dengue-immune monkeys to yellow fever virus. Amer. J. trop. Med. Hyg. **24**, 115—117 (1975).

THEILER, M., CASALS, J., MOUTOUSSES, C.: Etiology of the 1927—28 epidemic of dengue in Greece. Proc. Soc. exp. Biol. (N.Y.) **103**, 244—246 (1960).

THEILER, M., DOWNS, W. G.: The Arthropod-borne Viruses of Vertebrates, 578 pp. New Haven-London: Yale University Press 1973.

TIKASINGH, E. S., SPENCE, I., DOWNS, W. G.: The use of adjuvant and sarcoma 180 cells in the production of mouse hyperimmune ascitic fluids to arboviruses. Amer. J. trop. Med. Hyg. **15**, 219—226 (1966).

TODA, T., NAKAGAWA, Y.: Estimation of dengue virus particle size by human inoculation tests. Nippon Igaku **3332**, 877—878 (1943).

TODA, T., NAKAGAWA, Y.: Further studies on the particle size of dengue virus. Nippon Igaku **3368**, 302—303 (1944).

TODA, T., NAKAGAWA, Y., RYU, S.: Studies on dengue fever. III. Inoculation of dengue virus into the anterior chamber of the eye of rabbits. Nippon Igaku **3333**, 919—921 (1943).

TODA, T., NAKAGAWA, Y., SHITAMA, K.: Preservation of dengue virus by lyophilization (First Report). Nippon Igaku **3369**, 338—339 (1944).

TODA, T., NAKAGAWA, Y., SHITAMA, K., MISAO, T., KIMURA, M.: Preservation of dengue virus by lyophilization (Second Report). Rinsho & Kenkyu (Clinic and Research) **23**, 155—156 (1946).

TRENT, D. W., QUERSHI, A. A.: Structural and nonstructural proteins of St. Louis encephalitis virus. J. Virol. **7**, 379—388 (1971).

TSURUMI, S., SHIN, K.: Studies on dengue fever. I. Cultivation in fertilized chick embryos and inoculation into laboratory animals of the etiologic agent. Nippon Igaku **3341**, 1253—1255 (1943).

VENTURA, A. K., EHRENKRANZ, N. J., ROSENTHAL, D.: Placental passage of antibodies to dengue virus in persons living in a region of hyperendemic dengue virus infection. J. infect. Dis. **131** (Suppl.), S62—S68 (1975).

WERNER, G. H., SCHLESINGER, R. W.: Morphological and quantitative comparison between infectious and non-infectious forms of influenza virus. J. exp. Med. **100**, 203—216 (1954).

WESTAWAY, E. G.: Assessment and application of a cell line from pig kidney for plaque assay and neutralization tests with twelve group B arboviruses. Amer. J. Epidem. **84**, 439—456 (1966).

WESTAWAY, E. G.: Antibody responses in rabbits to the group B arbovirus Kunjin: Serologic activity of the fractionated immunoglobulins in homologous and heterologous reactions. J. Immunol. **100**, 569—580 (1968).

WESTAWAY, E. G.: Proteins specified by group B togaviruses in mammalian cells during productive infections. Virology **51**, 454—465 (1973).

WESTAWAY, E. G.: The proteins of Murray Valley encephalitis virus. J. gen. Virol. **27**, 283—292 (1975).

WESTAWAY, E. G., DELLA-PORTA, A. J., REEDMAN, B. M.: Specificity of IgM and IgG antibodies after challenge with antigenically related togaviruses. J. Immunol. **112**, 656—663 (1974).

WESTAWAY, E. G., SHEW, M., DELLA-PORTA, A. J.: Reactions of purified hemagglutinating antigens of flaviviruses with 19S and 7S antibodies. Infect. & Immun. **11**, 630—634 (1975).

WESTAWAY, E. G., REEDMAN, B. M.: Proteins of the group B arbovirus Kunjin. J. Virol. **4**, 688—693 (1969).

WHITEHEAD, R. H., CHAICUMPA, V., OLSON, L. C., RUSSELL, P. K.: Sequential dengue virus infections in the white-handed Gibbon *(Hylobates Lar)*. Amer. J. trop. Med. Hyg. **19**, 94—102 (1970).

WHO: Report of WHO Scientific Group. Arboviruses and Human Disease. WHO techn. Rep. Ser. No. 369, p. 9 (1967).

WHO REPORT: Pathogenic mechanisms in dengue haemorrhagic fever: Report of an international collaborative study. Bull. Wld Hlth Org. **48**, 117—133 (1973).

WIEBENGA, N. H.: The cultivation of dengue-1 (Hawaiian) virus in tissue culture I. Carrier culture of human skin cells infected with dengue-1 virus. Amer. J. Hyg. **73**, 350—364 (1961a).

WIEBENGA, N. J.: The cultivation of dengue-1 (Hawaiian) virus in tissue culture. II. Cytopathogenic virus subcultured from HuS 2806 dengue-1 carrier culture. Amer. J. Hyg. **73**, 365—377 (1961b).

WILDY, P.: Classification and nomenclature of viruses. First report of the International Committee on Nomenclature of Viruses. Monographs in Virology, Vol. 5, 81 pp. Basel: S. Karger 1971.

WINTER, P. E., NANTAPANICH, S., NISALAK, A., UDOMSAKDI, S., DEWEY, R. W., RUSSELL, P. K.: Recurrence of epidemic hemorrhagic fever in an insular setting. Amer. J. trop. Med. Hyg. 18, 573—579 (1969).

WINTER, P. E., SMITH, T. J., GOULD, D. J., NANTAPANICH, S., DEWEY, R. W., RUSSELL, P. K.: Dengue control on an Island in the Gulf of Thailand. III. Effect on transmission of dengue virus to man. Amer. J. trop. Med. Hyg. 20, 720—725 (1971).

WINTER, P. E., YUILL, T. M., UDOMSAKDI, S., GOULD, D., NANTAPANICH, S., RUSSELL, P.: An insular outbreak of dengue hemorrhagic fever. I. Epidemiological observations. Amer. J. trop. Med. Hyg. 17, 590—599 (1968).

WISSEMAN, C. L., JR.: The ecology of dengue: An addendum. In: Studies in Medical Geography (MAY, J. M., ed.), Vol. II, pp. 591—597. New York: Hafner Publishing Co. 1961.

WISSEMAN, C. L., JR.: Prophylaxis of dengue, with special reference to live virus vaccine. Proc. Jap. Soc. trop. Med. 7, 51—56 (1966).

WISSEMAN, C. L., JR., SWEET, B. H.: The ecology of dengue, Chapter 2. In: Studies in Medical Geography (MAY, J. M., ed.), Vol. II, pp. 15—40 and 504—515. New York: Hafner Publishing Co. 1961.

WISSEMAN, C. L., JR., SWEET, B. H.: Immunological studies with group B arthropod-borne viruses. III. Response of human subjects to revaccination with 17D strain yellow fever vaccine. Amer. J. trop. Med. Hyg. 11, 570—575 (1962).

WISSEMAN, C. L., JR., SWEET, B. H., KITAOKA, M., TAMIYA, T.: Immunological studies with group B arthropod-borne viruses. I. Broadened neutralizing antibody spectrum induced by strain 17D yellow fever vaccine in human subjects previously infected with Japanese encephalitis virus. Amer. J. trop. Med. Hyg. 11, 550—561 (1962).

WISSEMAN, C. L., JR., KITAOKA, M., TAMIYA, T.: Immunological studies with group B arthropod-borne viruses. V. Evaluation of cross-immunity against type 1 dengue fever in human subjects convalescent from subclinical natural Japanese encephalitis virus infection and vaccinated with 17D strain yellow fever vaccine. Amer. J. trop. Med. Hyg. 15, 588—599 (1966).

WISSEMAN, C. L., JR., SWEET, B. H., ROSENZWEIG, E. C., EYLAR, O. R.: Attenuated living type 1 dengue vaccines. Amer. J. trop. Med. Hyg. 12, 620—623 (1963).

YOSHINAKA, Y., HOTTA, S.: Purification of arboviruses grown in tissue culture. Proc. Soc. exp. Biol. (N.Y.) 137, 1047—1053 (1971).

YUILL, T. M., SUKHAVACHANA, P., NISALAK, A., RUSSELL, P. K.: Dengue-virus recovery by direct and delayed plaques in LLC-MK₂ cells. Amer. J. trop. Med. Hyg. 17, 441—448 (1968).

ZEBOVITZ, E., LEONG, J. K., DOUGHTY, S. C.: Japanese Encephalitis Virus replication: A procedure for the selective isolation and characterization of viral RNA species. Arch. ges. Virusforsch. 38, 319—327 (1972).

ZEBOVITZ, E., LEONG, J. K. L., DOUGHTY, S. C.: Involvement of the host cell nuclear envelope membranes in the replication of Japanese encephalitis virus. Infect. & Immun. 10, 204—211 (1974).

VIROLOGY MONOGRAPHS

VIROLOGY
MONOGRAPHS

VIROLOGY
MONOGRAPHS

Volume 15:

The Parvoviruses

By **G. Siegl**

1 figure. IV, 109 pages. 1976.

ISBN 3-211-81355-1 (Wien)
ISBN 0-387-81355-1 (New York)

Volume 16:

Dengue Viruses

By **R. W. Schlesinger**

34 figures. IV, 132 pages. 1977.

ISBN 3-211-81406-X (Wien)
ISBN 0-387-81406-X (New York)